1/13/16
$122.04

Total Hip Replacement Surgery
(Principles and Techniques)

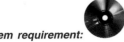

System requirement:
- **Windows XP or above**
- **Power DVD player (Software)**
- **Windows media player 10.0 version or above (Software)**

Accompanying DVD ROM is playable only in Computer and not in DVD player.

Kindly wait for few seconds for DVD to autorun. If it does not autorun then please do the following:
- Click on my computer
- Click the **CD/DVD drive** and after opening the drive, kindly double click the file **Jaypee**

DVD Contents

1. Surgical Technique Cemented Total Hip Replacement
2. Surgical Technique Cementless Total Hip Replacement

Total Hip Replacement Surgery
(Principles and Techniques)

SKS Marya

MS Orth (PGI), DNB Orth, MCh Orth (UK), FICS
Chairman, Orthopaedics and Institute of
Joint Replacement Surgery
Max Super Speciality Hospital, Saket
New Delhi, India

RK Bawari

MS Orth, DA
Consultant Orthopaedic Surgeon
Max Super Speciality Hospital, Saket
New Delhi, India

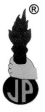

JAYPEE BROTHERS MEDICAL PUBLISHERS (P) LTD

New Delhi • St Louis (USA) • Panama City (Panama) • London (UK) • Ahmedabad
Bengaluru • Chennai • Hyderabad • Kochi • Kolkata • Lucknow • Mumbai • Nagpur

Published by
Jitendar P Vij
Jaypee Brothers Medical Publishers (P) Ltd

Corporate Office
4838/24 Ansari Road, Daryaganj, **New Delhi** - 110002, India, Phone: +91-11-43574357,
Fax: +91-11-43574314

Registered Office
B-3 EMCA House, 23/23B Ansari Road, Daryaganj, **New Delhi** - 110 002, India
Phones: +91-11-23272143, +91-11-23272703, +91-11-23282021
+91-11-23245672, Rel: +91-11-32558559, Fax: +91-11-23276490, +91-11-23245683
e-mail: jaypee@jaypeebrothers.com, Website: www.jaypeebrothers.com

Offices in India

- **Ahmedabad**, Phone: Rel: +91-79-32988717, e-mail: ahmedabad@jaypeebrothers.com
- **Bengaluru**, Phone: Rel: +91-80-32714073, e-mail: bangalore@jaypeebrothers.com
- **Chennai**, Phone: Rel: +91-44-32972089, e-mail: chennai@jaypeebrothers.com
- **Hyderabad**, Phone: Rel:+91-40-32940929, e-mail: hyderabad@jaypeebrothers.com
- **Kochi**, Phone: +91-484-2395740, e-mail: kochi@jaypeebrothers.com
- **Kolkata**, Phone: +91-33-22276415, e-mail: kolkata@jaypeebrothers.com
- **Lucknow**, Phone: +91-522-3040554, e-mail: lucknow@jaypeebrothers.com
- **Mumbai**, Phone: Rel: +91-22-32926896, e-mail: mumbai@jaypeebrothers.com
- **Nagpur**, Phone: Rel: +91-712-3245220, e-mail: nagpur@jaypeebrothers.com

Overseas Offices

- **North America Office, USA,** Ph: 001-636-6279734,
  e-mail: jaypee@jaypeebrothers.com, anjulav@jaypeebrothers.com
- **Central America Office, Panama City, Panama,** Ph: 001-507-317-0160,
  e-mail: cservice@jphmedical.com   Website: www.jphmedical.com
- **Europe Office, UK,** Ph: +44 (0) 2031708910, e-mail: dholman@jpmedical.biz; rfurn@jpmedical.biz;
  pheilbrunn@jpmedical.biz

Total Hip Replacement Surgery (Principles and Techniques)

This book has been published in good faith that the material provided by authors is original. Every effort is made to ensure accuracy of material, but the publisher, printer and authors will not be held responsible for any inadvertent error (s). In case of any dispute, all legal matters are to be settled under Delhi jurisdiction only.

First Edition: **2010**
ISBN 978-81-8448-884-5
Typeset at JPBMP typesetting unit
Printed at Sanat Printers, Kundli.

Dedicated to

My wife Mohini—my inspiration

SKS Marya

My wife Nidhi—for perpetual support and presence

RK Bawari

Preface

Why are we writing this book? Is there a dearth of material available on total hip replacement? Well, the idea first evolved during one of our basic Delhi arthroplasty courses. One of the participants observed that most of these meetings end up talking about hi-fi techniques and surgical accomplishments without much consideration towards the junior most surgeons.

We decided to produce basic books on total knee replacement and total hip replacement. This volume addresses some of the most simple and basic concerns of young or young at heart learners of the skill of arthroplasty.

Starting with an introduction, the history and evolution of hip replacement, the book goes on to talk about most aspects which a beginner would want to understand and many times find it difficult to question a senior surgeon for the fear of being ridiculed or embarrassed.

Live surgical videos of cemented and cementless hip replacement have been provided with this volume. The technique has been kept to the most simple demonstration and it is hoped that the learners would identify with the commentary.

A chapter on complications has been added to make the readers aware and cautious keeping in mind that principle of "What the mind does not know, the eyes cannot see."

Last but not the least, a small write up on newer advances in hip arthroplasty should excite the readers to dig deep into the vast literature available on this topic.

SKS Marya
RK Bawari

Acknowledgment

A few pictures have been taken from the Johnson and Johnson website and the authors are grateful for the same.

Contents

Chapter One

Hip Replacement— History and Evolution

Hip arthroplasty started in the beginning of the twentieth century with the procedure of contouring and interpositional-layer insertion between the articulating bony surfaces at the hip (*Interpositional arthroplasty*) (Fig. 1.1). Corrective osteotomy of the proximal femur was simultaneously done for fixed deformities, e.g. ankylosis of the hip joint. Osteotomy alone was the only procedure available before this to treat such conditions. Sir Robert Jones (1912) used gold foil as an interpositional layer. Murphy (1915) combined osteotomy with interposition of soft tissue at the hip. Other materials used for the purpose at that time include fascia lata, chromicised pig bladder, skin, etc. However, all had uniformly unsuccessful results.

Smith-Petersen in 1923 introduced the concept of *mould arthroplasty* (Fig. 1.2) as an alternative to interpositional membrane. This was based on his chance discovery of synovial tissue formation around an impregnated glass-piece in the thigh of a patient. The idea was to put in a mould of an inert material between the freshened surfaces of the femoral head and acetabulum, which would guide nature's repair to form smooth articulating surfaces. The implant could be removed once such surfaces were formed. Glass moulds were too fragile. Alternative materials like Bakelite Viscalloid and Pyrex were attempted, which were not very durable either. Besides, these materials induced severe foreign body reaction and bone destruction. Because of high failure the procedure had to be abandoned.

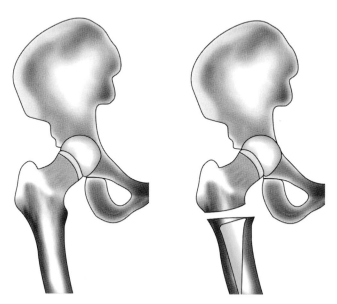

Fig. 1.1: *Interpositional arthroplasty*: Interpositional arthroplasty was used with or without osteotomy to correct ankylosis and painful hip conditions. Interposition of different materials was done to prevent recurrence of bone growth and maintain motion. Tissues of various types were tried by various surgeons: Ollier (1885)- soft tissue; Murphy (1902)- fascia lata; Loewe (1913)-skin; Baer (1918)- Pig's bladder

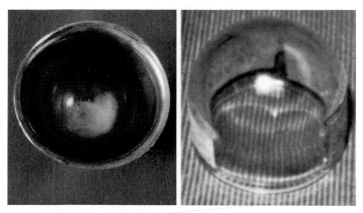

Fig. 1.2: *Mould arthroplasty:* Smith-Petersen and others tried putting a mould of inert material between the articular surfaces of the hip joint viz. Glass (1923), Pyrex (1933), Bakelite (1937) and Vitalium (1938). It proved that the acetabulum will tolerate a foreign body

In 1938 Smith-Petersen used *Vitallium* an alloy of cobalt, chromium and molybdenum used by dentists to line the raw bony surfaces (*cup arthroplasty*) (Fig. 1.3). This was found to be a suitable material. It was a kind of hemi-surface arthroplasty of the hip. Cup arthroplasty and later Aufranc's modification of the same was the standard for hip reconstruction at that time. However only about one half of the cup arthroplasties relieved pain successfully. It was not possible to replace bony deficiencies or correct bony abnormalities or shortening with this procedure. Though it was not a stable fixation and the outcomes were unpredictable some survived for many years.

Phillip Wiles (1938, London), was the first to attempt metal-on-metal (Figs 1.4 and 1.6) articulation. He used a stainless steel cup with spikes for the acetabulum. The femoral head was resurfaced with a stainless steel shell, which was fixed with an inter-trochanteric device to the side-plate on the shaft of femur. AT Moore credited Bohlman for use of a cobalt-chrome ball fitted to a Smith-Petersen nail in 1939. In early 1940's Moore and Bohlman replaced the upper end of femur in a patient with a 12-inch steel prosthesis. In 1946, the Judet brothers, used an endoprosthesis with a femoral head of acrylic attached through an acrylic stem. Because of severe wear the acrylic was changed to a metal (cobalt-chrome) alloy.

In 1950's Moore and Thompson individually developed stemmed metal prosthesis. This was the beginning of *hemiarthroplasty* (Fig. 1.5). Both Thompson's and Moore's metallic implants were unipolar prostheses with long stems (endoprosthesis) that allowed transmission of weight-bearing forces along the axis of the femoral shaft, unlike the previous designs (which generated high shear forces on the short stem placed within the femoral neck). The Moore prosthesis was fenestrated to permit bone growth. Thompson's prosthesis was without any fenestration and was also cemented once bone cement became available. These prostheses have worked very well; they are still in use with little modification. These

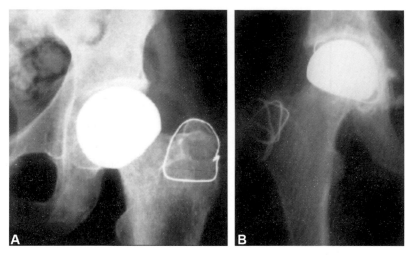

Figs 1.3A and B: *Cup arthroplasty*: (A) A hemi-surface replacement, (B) Smith-Petersen double cup-a metal surface replacement femoral component and a polymer acetabular component

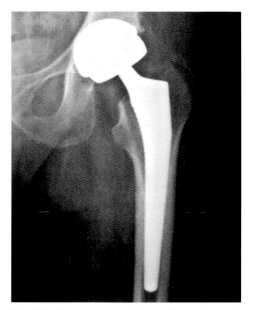

Fig. 1.4: *Metal-on-metal hip prosthesis*: X-ray of metal-on-metal cementless hip, note the large bearing size

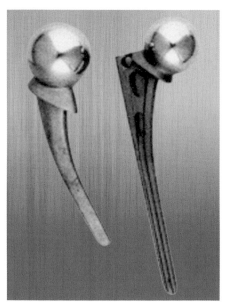

Fig. 1.5: *Unipolar femoral components*: 1950–Thompson Prosthesis: Large head and collared curved intramedullary stem. 1952–Moore Prosthesis: Large head and collared long straight cementless stem with fenestrations for bone in growth

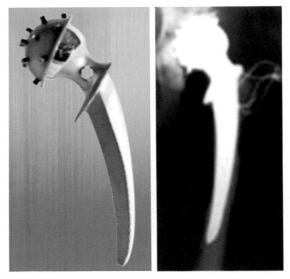

Fig. 1.6: *McKee-Farrar prosthesis*: McKee Farrar metal on metal hip prosthesis had a high initial failure due to poor neck, stem design and improper orientation of the implants. Also the concept of peri-operative asepsis was not established leading to high infection rate

have press-fit fixation however may produce varying degrees of femoral bone loss. There may also be delayed erosion of bone on the pelvic side; that highlighted the need to resurface the acetabulum.

Kenneth McKee modified metal-on-metal (MOM) arthroplasty in 1950's. He introduced cobalt-chrome alloy articulations. Thompson-type stem of femoral implant was designed. Watson-Farrar modified the neck to reduce impingement. McKee modified the acetabulum, for cement fixation. The first series of McKee–Farrar total hip replacement (Fig. 1.6) (1956 to 1960) had a high incidence of failure. The bearing combination of MOM was suspected to be unfavorable and the cause of failure, which, we now know is not true. The failure was due to poor designing and implant placement besides non-availability of antibiotic prophylaxis and poor aseptic techniques. Some of these prostheses have functioned over 20 years. KM Sivash (Moscow, 1950's), Peter Ring (England,1964) and others designed their versions of all-metal prosthesis (Fig. 1.7).

Sir John Charnley is credited as the 'father of total hip arthroplasty' for his pioneering work in all aspects of total hip arthroplasty, including the concept of 'low frictional torque arthroplasty', lubrication, materials, design, trochanteric osteotomy, asepsis and operating room hygiene. His other major contribution was the use of polymethylmethacrylate (PMMA), a cold-curing acrylic cement for fixation of the prosthetic components.

Charnley attributed the squeak heard in patients with a Judet prosthesis to marked friction between the acrylic head and the acetabulum. This led to enough torque on the implants to loosen up the fixation on the respective bones. He confirmed the low coefficient of friction of a normal joint in the presence of joint fluid. He realised that in joint replacement

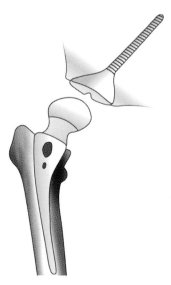

Fig. 1.7: *Peter Ring prosthesis*: Ring's prosthesis matched with Moore's stem was a metal-on-metal articulation. A high incidence of failure was reported due to breakage of the threaded stem on the acetabular component at its base

the articulating surfaces are subjected to boundary lubrication. He also determined that the coefficient of friction of a steel ball against polytetrafluoroethylene (PTFE/Teflon) was close to that of a normal joint. Between 1958 and 1963 he had developed and tried various types of prosthetic hips. He inserted large head Thompson stem and lined the acetabulum with PTFE shell. Charnley fixed the stem of the femoral prosthesis securely with PMMA bone cement. This permitted more uniform transfer of stress to a larger bone surface. In 1961 he realized that "the best engineering practice would be to use the smallest diameter ball which could cope with the expected load". By trial and error the right size determined was 22.225 mm (7/8 inch). This decreased the resistance to movement by reducing the moment (lever arm) of the frictional force. He realized that with a larger head the pressure per unit of surface was less and that this would tend to reduce wear. However, he still considered it more important to reduce frictional torque and to have a cup with a thick wall. He continued using press-fit PTFE shell for a long time. PTFE shells wore off faster and were replaced with high-density polyethylene (HDPE) and later by ultrahigh molecular weight polyethylene (UHMWPE). Though the initial cementing of these cups was suspect it was eventually realized to be holding very well and from 1966 onwards UHMWPE cemented cups were the standard implants. The procedure of cementing, use of 22.225 mm diameter head metal on polyethylene articulation and trochanteric osteotomy together form the concept of '**low frictional torque arthroplasty (LFA) (Fig. 1.8).**' Charnley had earlier attempted resurfacing the femoral head but abandoned this procedure because of high incidence of what he proposed was avascular necrosis of the head.

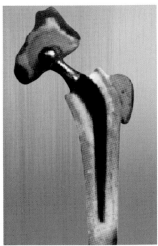

Fig. 1.8: Charnley principles of THR (LFA)

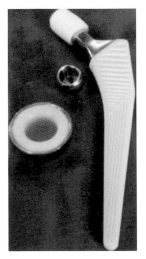

Fig. 1.9: *Bipolar hip prosthesis*: Components of modular bipolar hip with a cementless stem. The parts are assembled on the patient's body. The length of inner-head can be adjusted to the requirement. The outer head corresponds to the patient's natural femoral head size

In an attempt to decrease the acetabular wear with the traditional endoprosthesis for hemiarthroplasty McKeever and Collision developed bipolar endoprosthesis in the 1950's. The idea was to achieve more movement between the prosthetic components than between the metal and the acetabulum. Gilberty and Bateman individually developed the current generation of bipolar hips. Despite the initial expectations the benefit of bipolar prosthesis over unipolar implant has been debated, (Fig. 1.9).

Charnley first used methylmethacrylate to cement the femoral component in 1958. The basic concept of bone cement fixation still holds true. The commercial cast sheets of polymethylmethacrylate (Plexiglas), in the early 1930's, led to its development as a denture material. The original material was molded under heat and pressure. In 1936 it was discovered that a mixture of methylmethacrylate monomer and ground polymer produced moldable dough in the presence of benzoyl peroxide. In subsequent years polymer beads were added to improve mouldability. In the year 1943 it was discovered that the dough could be polymerized at room temperature if dimethyl-p-toludine was added with benzoyl peroxide. This was routinely used in 1940's for dentures and cranioplasty prosthesis. Though Judet brothers and others had used PMMA, nobody had used it as a means to stabilize the prosthetic implant. In 1958 Charnley operated on the first case at Manchester where bone cement was used to completely fill the medullary canal to adapt to the bony interface thereby facilitating stress transfer, in turn stabilizing and anchoring the prosthesis. Cementing technique has long evolved since then. This includes use of injectable low-viscosity bone cement, occlusion of medullary stem, reduction of porosity by centrifuging, pressurization of cement and centralization of the stem.

Sir John Charnley's concept of metal on polyethylene articulation and use of small diameter head has overshadowed the field of hip replacement for a long time. However, the major drawback with it is the excessive polyethylene wear and the consequent osteolysis, aseptic loosening and implant failure. This is even more pronounced with prostheses having larger diameter heads which were designed in an attempt to improve hip stability. All this led to research for alternative

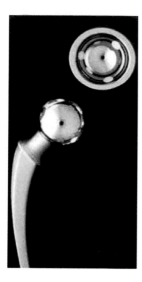

Fig. 1.10: Original metal-on-metal Müller prosthesis

bearing surfaces. Metal-on-metal (MOM) ceramic-on-polyethylene (COP), ceramic on ceramic (COC) and ceramic-on-metal (COM) articulations are few such options.

MOM surface replacement is a direct descendant of cup arthroplasty. Muller (1967) introduced the first generation metal-on-metal surface arthroplasty. This was a press fit design and had excellent preliminary result. He also designed stemmed MOM prostheses at the same time (Fig. 1.10). Though the initial results were satisfactory, he moved on to metal-on-polyethylene articulations. The results of hip resurfacing in the 1970s and 1980s were disappointing and the procedure was almost abandoned.

The credit of revival of metal-on metal articulations goes to Bernard G. Weber in collaboration with the erstwhile 'Sulzer Orthopedics' (Switzerland), 1988. This was due to the availability of the low-wear, high-carbon metal bearings of Co-Cr-Mo alloy (Metasul). The second generation metal-on-metal total hip arthroplasty was launched using 28 mm heads. The low wear and added stability and good range of motion were encouraging. It was noted that every one-millimeter increase in head size yielded approximately one-degree increase in range of motion. The introduction of hard cobalt-chromium alloy led to the designing of thinner acetabular implants which could accommodate correspondingly larger femoral heads. The second generation metal-on-metal surface arthroplasty evolved with the use of the arthroplasty system developed by Heinz Wagner (Germany) and Derek McMinn (England) individually in 1991. Amstutz (1996) developed the Conserve Hip Resurfacing (USA). Two designs, Cormet resurfacing hip system and the Birmingham hip resurfacing evolved from the McMinn system in 1997. These third generation MOM surface replacements were better in terms of designing and metallurgy. Durom Hip (Zimmer, Switzerland, 2001), Articular Surface Replacement (ASR™; DePuy, UK, 2003) (Figs 1.11A and B) and others are reportedly the fourth generation metal-on-metal articular surface replacements. These are bone conserving surgeries, use Co-Cr-Mo alloy bearing with high

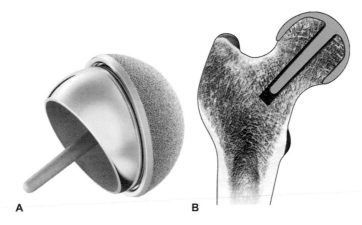

A   **B**

Figs 1.11A and B: *Surface replacement arthroplasty:* (A) ASR™ Hip (J&J, DePuy), (B) Surface replacement is a bone conserving surgery for the hip permitting large range of motion. However careful patient selection is mandatory for favorable long term result

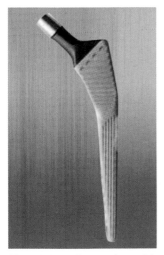

Fig. 1.12: *Cementless hip prosthesis:* Corail™ stem (J&J, DePuy) is a titanium stem with HA coating. The prosthesis has shown remarkable long term survivorship

carbon content, have cementless fixation of the acetabular component and the femoral component is cemented.

COC and ceramic on polyethylene (COP) modular hips are gaining attention again. Zirconia is a newer ceramic which is less prone to fractures. The ceramics exist in oxidized state and unlike metal articulations are not prone to oxidative damage in the body. Some studies have documented less wear of plastic cups with ceramic heads as compared to metal ones. Ceramic on metal hip is the latest addition. Ceramics are expensive implants.

As loosening and osteolysis on the bone-cement interface is a frequent complication with cemented implants the cementless fixation has come into vogue again. The current designs may be press-fit, porous-coated and hydroxyapatite-coated (HA-coated) surfaces (Fig. 1.12). These use the principles of bone in-growth and on-growth as a means of achieving long-lasting skeletal fixation. Though the prospects look good not all designs have similar success reports. These may be due to inadequate initial fixation (a mandatory prerequisite) and excessive particle induced osteolysis. With time certain design parameters have been realized to be important for cementless fixation. Good quality, 'super alloys' have been discovered which have resulted in negligible breakage of the stem (Figs 1.13A and B).

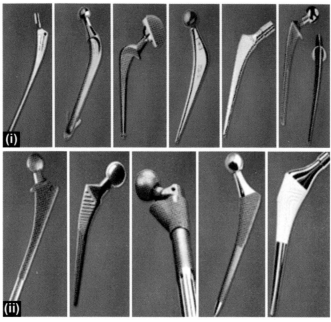

Fig. 1.13A: *Various hip prosthesis*: Femoral components (i) Cemented femoral designs, (ii) Cementless femoral designs

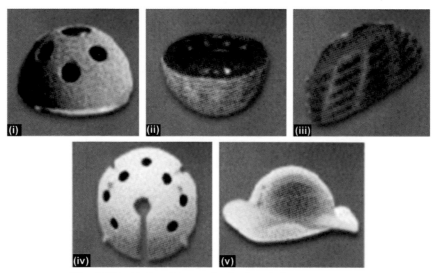

Fig. 1.13B: *Various hip prosthesis*: Acetabular components—
(i-iv) cementless and (v) cemented

Modular hip systems have evolved reducing the inventory of stock. These allow better balance of limb length and stability. They also add to the versatility of articulation and stem choice on the operating table. Smaller hip designs (mini-hip) are becoming popular in younger patients which allow easier revisions.

Chapter Two

Implants Systems and Designs—Options Today

Hip replacement has evolved significantly in the past two decades (Fig. 2.1). A whole array of design options are available to choose from (Fig. 2.2). Companies have come up with various options, for the acetabular and femoral components in terms of material, design, size of the implant, surface finish, type of fixation, etc. However, none of these can be said to be more superior or inferior, though certain implants may have more advantage in a selected situation. Herein comes the role of the orthopedic surgeon—in making the right decision and therefore a thorough knowledge of the options is essential.

The surgery may be a conventional total hip replacement, hemi-replacement or a surface replacement where-in indicated. The acetabulum may be cemented polyethylene socket or cementless press-fit socket, with or without screws. The cementless cup may be a monobloc metal implant or may have a liner. The liner may be made up of polyethylene, metal, polyethylene backed metal or ceramic. The femoral stems, may also be cemented or cementless. The cemented stem may be with a regular finish or a polished taper finish. The cementless stem may be fabricated of cobalt-chromium alloy, titanium or composites. These may be press fit, with or without macro interlock or may be porous coated. The porous coated implants may be extensively porous coated or proximally coated. The surface treatment may include sintered beads, plasma spray, titanium fiber metal and corundmization with or without hydroxyapatite (HA) coating. The femoral head and neck may be a part of the monobloc stem or, more commonly are modular components. The femoral head size may be as large as the normal contralateral hip 36 mm, 28 mm or 22.225 mm sized Charnley's hip. The modular head may be metal or ceramic.

Total hip femoral and acetabular components with their respective assemblies/instrumentation are commonly referred to as a 'total hip system'.

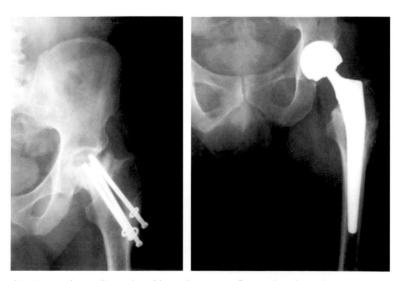

Fig. 2.1: Pre and postoperative radiographs—hip replacement. Cementless large bearing metal on metal hip for avascular necrosis of femoral head in a patient with fracture neck of femur with failed screw fixation

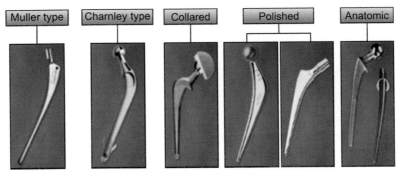

Fig. 2.2A: Cemented stem designs

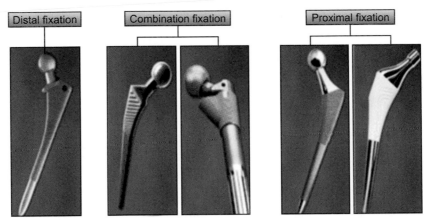

Fig. 2.2B: Cementless stem designs

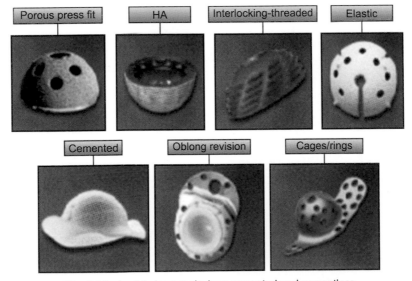

Fig. 2.2C: Acetabular cup designs-cemented and cementless

Fixation of Implants (Fig. 2.3)

- *Cemented:* Where both the acetabular and femoral components are fixed with bone cement
- *Cementless*: Where both the acetabular and femoral components are fixed by virtue of their design and surface finish, without the use of bone cement.
- *Hybrid*: A combination of the previous two; where either of the side is cemented and the other is cementless.

Cementless fixation is initially achieved by pressfit and subsequently by in-growth and/or on-growth of bone on the implant. The bone and the implant then form one continous unit.

The in-growth is achieved by using porous metal coating over the stem and the outer surface of the cup. The porous metals used are:

- Cobalt-chrome powder or beads attached by sintering or
- Titanium beads or wire-mesh (commercially pure titanium- cpTi) attached by diffusion bonding.

Both materials have proved to be satisfactory so far. Titanium femoral stems has been recommended by many designers because of its superior biocompatibility, high fatigue strength, and lower modulus of elasticity which is closer to that of the bone. However, titanium is more notch-sensitive predisposing it to initiation of cracks through metallurgical defects and at sites of poor attachment of porous coatings, particularly on the tensile surface.

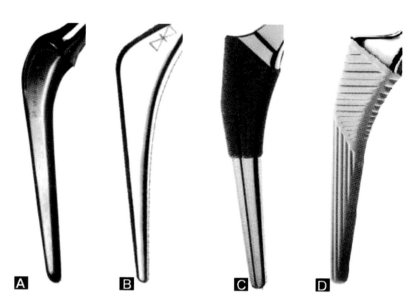

Figs. 2.3A to D: *Surface finish of femoral implants*: Surface finish of implant varies from (A) non-polished (Charnley prosthesis), (B) polished (C-stem) in case of cemented implants. The cementless implants have a coating of metal mesh or sintered beads which may be (C) proximally coated or fully coated for in-growth of bone. This may also be (D) HA coated for bony on-growth

Multiple layers of pore-forming material about 800 μm (300 μm-1 mm) in thickness are used to create interconnected open pores with surface topography of recesses and outcroppings for in-growth of bone. 30% to 60% porosity calculated on a volume basis is ideally required. Pore sizes differ markedly in the commercially available brands:

- Porocoat surface (DePuy, Warsaw, Ind.)—150 to 350 μm
- PCA (Stryker, Howmedica, East Rutherford, NJ)—400 to 1200 μm
- Titanium wire mesh system (Zimmer, Warsaw, Ind.)—an average of 280 μm.

Large pores especially on the tensile surface will act as a stress riser and may lead to implant failure.

Plasma-spraying of ceramics—Hydroxyapatite (HA) and Tricalcium phosphate (TCP) over cpTi or Ti alloy substrates is a method of achieving biological fixation by on-growth. HA converts to other forms of ceramic such as TCP which are bio-active as a result of partial dissolution. This layer is typically 50 μm thick.

Implants with irregular or textured surface have also been tried for press-fit cementless fixation.

Stability by in-growth of bone is achieved by mechanical interlock of bone on implant-osseointegration. However there are certain pre-requisites for cement-less fixation to succeed:

- Secure press-fit as initial fixation
- Limited early loading: maximum tolerable relative displacement is 50 μm
- Pore size more than or equal to 100 μm.
- Adequate vascularity.

FEMORAL COMPONENTS

The role of the femoral prosthesis is the replacement of the femoral head and neck of the arthritic, fractured or necrotic hip with a stable component that carefully re-establishes the intra-capsular femoral length with proper offset. The aim of replacement is a biomechanically sound and stable hip joint. The hip systems in current use achieve fixation of the femoral prosthesis with an intramedullary metal stem. The selection of femoral implant is based not only on the requirements of the articulating surface but also on the requirements of stem fixation. The fixation alternatives may hence be cemented or cementless. Cementless stems in turn may be with porous surface for in-growth with or without HA or other ceramic coating for ongrowth; or press-fit varieties.

Cemented Femoral Stems

Cemented stems (Fig. 2.4) became the standard for femoral component fixation after the introduction of acrylic cement by Charnley in the early 1960's. These have had excellent long-term survivorship. Certain material and design features of cemented stems have been found to be useful. These are fabricated of high-strength superalloys like cobalt-chrome alloy (with higher modulus of elasticity) which reduces stresses within the proximal cement mantle and also the resulting incidence of fracture of the bone cement. The preferred cross section of the stem is a broad medial border and broader lateral border to load the proximal

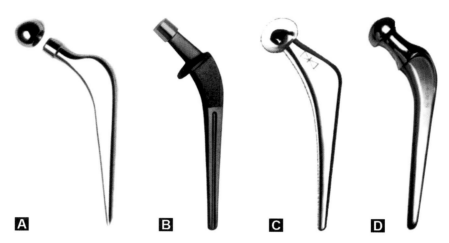

Figs. 2.4A to D: *Cemented femoral stems*: (A) Exeter Hip- Double tapered highly polished stem, (B) Spectron EF- Grit blast proximal third with proximal collar, (C) C-stem – Triple tapered highly polished stem, (D) Charnley stem- Monobloc implant

cement mantle in compression. Designs with sharp edges are avoided as these may initiate fracture in the cement mantle. Noncircular cross-section such as a rounded rectangle or an ellipse, with or without surface grooves or a longitudinal slots improve rotational stability of the stem within the cement mantle. In a collared design the length of the implant to be inserted while cementing is pre-determined. They make visualization of cement mantle difficult at the time of implant removal when doing revision surgeries.

Stems may have a polished dull or matte finish. Polished stems were found to have longer life and are preferred. A variety of collarless tapered stem with polished finish have been known to have performed very well e.g. Exeter^{TM} stem and C-stem^{TM}. Though this allows a small amount of subsidence it maintains compressive stresses within the cement mantle. The cemented stems may be monobloc or modular. The common designs are:
• Charnley stem
• Polished tapered stems
• Collared type.

Despite the current popularity of cement-less fixation cement is likely to remain an attractive option for fixation of femoral component in the foreseeable future.

Cementless Femoral Stems

The currently available porous coated stems include a wide variety of designs which may be monobloc or modular. The option of alloy used may be cobalt-chrome, titanium or composite. The surface treatment may be sintered beads, titanium mesh, etc. with or without HA coating (Fig. 2.5). Anatomical studies of femoral endosteal geometry suggest that exact fit of a prosthesis within the cortex is not possible because of large variations in anatomy

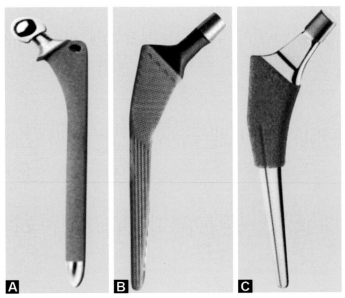

Figs. 2.5A to C: *Cementless femoral stems:* (A) Solution stem, (B) Corail™ stem (J&J, DePuy) fully coated stem with HA coating, (C) M/L Taper proximally coated stem

and age-related changes in the diameter of the canal. However, if the load is transferred over a large area, with emphasis on certain priority areas of contact, the normal strain patterns of the femur will be better achieved, favoring long-term fixation. The femur must be machined to a greater degree to accept a cementless stem. Although the extent of porous coating necessary remains controversial, most agree that porous coating should be circumferential at its proximal extent. The cementless stems may be:

• Extensively porous coated stem
• Proximal in-growth stem:
  – Tapered stem
  – Cylindrical stem.

Extensively porous coated stems achieve initial stability by diaphyseal fixation. These designs are not preferred by some authors as these may cause proximal stress-shielding leading to thigh pain and are also more difficult to remove in subsequent revision surgery, if needed. *Some systems have modular design for better proximal and distal fit (e.g. S-ROM™ system Depuy).*

Proximal ingrowth stems have coated surface for in-growth only in the proximal metaphyseal part. These reportedly have a lesser incidence of thigh pain as weight transfer is through the metaphysis. The design may be double tapered stem or cylindrical stem. The tapered stem has a cross-sectional anatomy which is two or three dimensionally tapered along the entire length of the prosthesis depending on the design. These are usually tapered titanium stems distally that progressively form a bulky segment proximally. The tapered

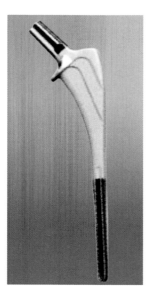

Fig. 2.6: *Collared femoral component.* Mallory-Head collared prosthesis (Biomet)

stem establishes bony contact in the metaphyseal region. If the initial contact is not satisfactory it will subside to a newer level to reestablish bony contact. This permits proximal loading. The cylindrical stem on the other hand has cross-sectional anatomy which is two or three dimensionally tapered proximally but is a cylinder in the diaphyseal portion.

The cementless femoral stems may be:
- Anatomical (right or left).
- Straight.

The anatomic stems with in-built neck version are side specific. These incorporate a posterior bow in the metaphyseal portion and variably an anterior bow in the diaphyseal portion, corresponding to the geometry of the femoral canal. The non-anatomic (straight) stems can be used on either side.

The collared prosthesis prevents subsidence however may not permit satisfactory fixation in all the cases (Fig. 2.6).

ACETABULAR COMPONENTS

Correct acetabular cup placement is essential for reestablishment of the center of the hip joint. The version and inclination of the prosthetic cup should be appropriate. The cemented prosthesis should be seated in correct alignment in the first place itself as it cannot be modified. The cementless cups on the other hand can be reoriented if desired, also these have modular liners that allow minor correction in its orientation.

Cemented Acetabular Component

The cemented sockets are thick-walled polyethylene cups (Fig. 2.7). Vertical and horizontal grooves on the external surface increase stability within the cement mantle, wire rings (markers) on the plastic allow better assessment of position on postoperative radiographs. Newer designs with PMMA spacers typically 3 mm in height, ensure a uniform cement mantle and avoid the phenomenon of 'bottoming out' which results in a thin or discontinuous cement mantle at the summit of the cup. Other designs have a flange at the rim of the component that can be cut to suit the size of the acetabulum. It helps in achieving even pressurization of the cement and also prevents 'bottoming out'.

Cemented fixation is satisfactory in elderly, low-demand patients because of simplicity and low cost of polyethylene components.

Cemented acetabular fixation also is used in some tumor reconstructions and when operative circumstances indicate that bone ingrowth into a porous surface is unlikely, as in revision arthroplasty in which extensive acetabular bone grafting has been necessary. In these instances, a cemented acetabular component is often used with an acetabular reinforcement ring (Fig. 2.8).

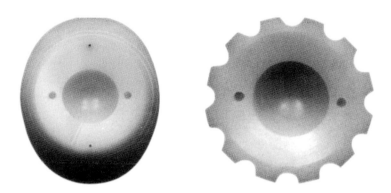

Fig. 2.7: Cemented acetabular components

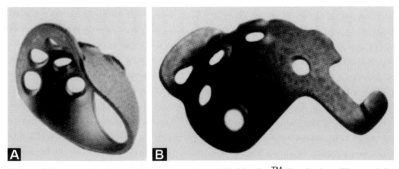

Figs. 2.8A and B: *Acetabular reinforcement rings*: (A) Mueller™ Roof ring (Zimmer) for simple revision cases, (B) Reinforcement Ring with Hook15 for moderate revision cases. These are available in various sizes

Cementless Acetabular Components (Press-fit/ in-growth Sockets)

Cementless acetabular components are porous coated over the entire outer surface (Fig. 2.9). Fixation of the porous shell may be augmented with transacetabular screws. Certain designs have pegs and spikes to enhance stability. Other cups have enlarged rim at the periphery for equatorial fixation. The shells may be HA coated for bony on-growth. These are available in various sizes (40 mm to 70 mm). The liner used may be made up of polyethylene, metal or ceramic. The outer diameter of the liner matches the shell and the inner diameter is selected according to the femoral head size chosen (22 mm, 28 mm, 32 mm etc). The liner is usually fixed to the shell by a snap-fit mechanism. Polyethylene liners with offset have been used to provide greater superior and posterior coverage. These compensate for any incorrect shell orientation planned or erroneous. In superior acetabular deficiency the shell may be placed vertical and compensated with a liner with postero-superior overhang. Back side wear is a known complication of the cementless acetabular components and may lead to osteolysis, loosening and subsidence.

Bipolar Acetabular Components

The bipolar prosthesis consists of polished metal femoral head which mates with a locking polyethylene bearing which in turn has a polished metal cup seated on it (Fig. 2.10). The outer metal cup is of the size of the anatomical femoral head. There is motion between both the mating surfaces viz. the inner head and the polyethylene liner; and the outer metal cup and the natural acetabular cartilage. The axis of polyethylene and metallic cup is eccentric thus on loading the two move separately allowing greater motion without jeopardizing hip stability and minimizing damage to the normal acetabular cartilage. There is however, some debate about the actual motion between the two surfaces.

MATERIALS AND BEARING SURFACES

Biomaterials commonly used in total hip arthroplasty are metals, polyethylene, ceramics and PMMA. The approximate modulus of elasticity of cement, bone, and orthopedic metals are in easy ratios - 2 (PMMA): 20 (bone): 100 (titanium): 200 (stainless steel and cobalt

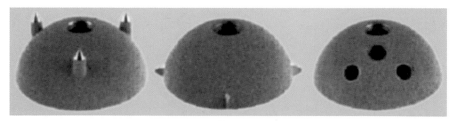

Fig. 2.9: *Cementless acetabular component*: Duraloc ™ (J&J, DePuy) series of cementless cups with various options of fixation. These include spikes, peripheral fins and holes for screw fixation. These are titanium implants with surface of sintered beads for bony ingrowth

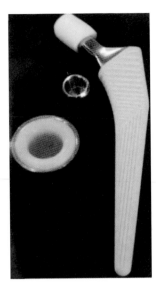

Fig. 2.10: *Bipolar hip components:* Corail™ cementless stem with modular head neck and outer bipolar Hasting head with polyethylene liner to match with the patient size

alloys). Titanium is 5 times stiffer than the bone however it is still the closest to the bone in stiffness when compared to other metals.

Metals

Metal alloys currently in use in orthopedics are:
- Cobalt-based alloys
- Titanium and titanium-based alloys
- Stainless steel
- Others, e.g. Zirconium, tantulum, combination metals.

Cobalt-based Alloys

Cast cobalt-chromium-molybdenum (Co-Cr-Mo) alloy has the longest and the maximum use in the history of arthroplasty. It has excellent wear and corrosion resistance, acceptable biocompatibility and satisfactory fatigue strength. Toughness is adequate (i.e. strength is high). However the casting process can produce large grain size in-homogeneities and porosities. These pores particularly in areas of high tensile stress can become stress-risers and lead to implant fracture. Modern techniques such as mold inoculation, forging, hot isostatic pressing have been introduced which greatly reduce grain size and porosities.

High carbon cobalt-based alloys are good materials for manufacturing bearing surfaces of implants. Co-Cr alloys are also used to make structural component such as a femoral stem (cemented).

Titanium and Titanium-based Alloys

Titanium (Ti) and titanium-based alloys are more resistant to corrosion in a chloride environment of body fluids compared to both stainless steel and cobalt alloys. Its protective oxide surface is highly inert and reforms easily after damage. The modulus of elasticity is about half that of stainless steel and cobalt alloys which is favorable as it allows load transfer to the bone, particularly in cement-less fixation. However the same fact deters its use in cemented hip arthroplasty as there is an increased load on the PMMA mantle leading to cement fracture. The Ti alloys commonly used are Ti_6Al_4V, TiAlNb and unalloyed commercially pure titanium (cpTi). Ti_6Al_4V is machinable. Surface defect, if any, has a greater tendency to propogate and fracture the prosthesis with titanium compared to cobalt–chrome alloy. Commercially pure titanium is used to make titanium beads or mesh coatings on cementless Ti stems for bone in-growth. Both titanium based alloys form a more intimate bond with bone than cobalt alloys.

Titanium-based alloys are not good bearing materials because of their low wear-resistance and a high coefficient of friction. Newer techniques like nitriding and nitrogen ion implantation, have been shown to increase surface hardness.

Titanium is used for manufacturing cementless femoral stems and acetabular shells.

Stainless Steel

Stainless steel is inferior to both cobalt and titanium alloys in terms of corrosion resistance, biocompatibility, and fatigue life. Also there is no current satisfactory method for applying a porous surface to stainless steel for bone in-growth.

Combination Metals

Cobalt alloys can be used with titanium alloys, e.g. Ti femoral stem with modular cobalt-chrome head. Also each type of alloy—stainless steel, cobalt, and titanium—can be mated with other alloy of the same type. Cobalt alloy and stainless steel used together will corrode the stainless steel implant, similarly titanium alloy should not be combined with stainless steel.

Plastics in Hip Arthroplasty

PTFE (Teflon) was initially used by Sir John Charnley. This had poor wear properties. HDPE (High density PE) used subsequently had similarly dismal wear rate. The next generation of plastics was UHMWPE (Ultra high molecular weight PE). UHMWPE are longest, least-branched chain of molecules of PE produced under low-pressure. Wear particles produced persist indefinitely in the body and induce severe osteolysis. Therefore a need for tougher plastics was felt which led to the development of highly cross-linked UHMWPE (XLPE).

XLPE are long PE chains cross linked to each other that have remarkable resistance to both wear and oxidative degradation. The acetabular cups or liners for MOP (metal-on-polyethylene) total hip arthroplasties are made of UHMWPE and XLPE. These plastics are chemically inert with good resistance to creep (i.e., slow, permanent deformation in the direction of stress).

PE components (acetabular liners in hips) are manufactured either by:

a. Extrusion (machining of extruded bar stock made up of UHMWPE which are in turn made up from PE powder),

b. Hot molding (compression molded from PE powder directly into the desired shapes close to the final dimensions, with little subsequent machining).

These are then subjected to high doses of radiation (gamma or electron beam radiation at 5 to 15 M rad) which produces PE with a highly cross-linked molecular structure. This happens due to formation of free radicals which lead to oxidation of the molecular chains. However, when these were subsequently exposed to air at implantation led to early degradation of the plastic. These free radicals are therefore now removed by annealing, i.e. melting the plastic again at approximately 150°C. The implants are finally packed and sterilized. Sterilization may be done with 2.5 M rad of gamma or electron radiation in an inert environment (nitrogen gas or vacuum). Ethylene oxide (EtO) or Gas Plasma with ionized gases are other options. However the latter two lead to surface sterilization only.

Autoclaving plastic components has no role as it brings about permanent change in shape and leads to degradation of the material due to the high temperature and pressure.

Ceramics

Ceramics used in hip arthroplasty are aluminum oxide (alumina) and zirconium oxide (zirconia) (Fig. 2.11). These are produced by consolidating the small grains either by *sintering* (holding a low-density aggregate of powder particles at a temperature below its melting point until the particles grow and fuse into each other) or by *hot pressing* (applying pressure and heat to speed the densification process).

Ceramic components are chemically inert, do not undergo oxidative wear, do not decompose nor produce metal ions. These are far stronger and less brittle under compression than in tension. Ceramics are hard hence can be polished to very smooth surfaces. They have less abrasive-wear. They make good bearing surfaces. The coefficient of friction of COC (ceramic-on ceramic), COP (ceramic on polyethylene) is lower than MOP and the wear is reportedly 3 to 16 times less.

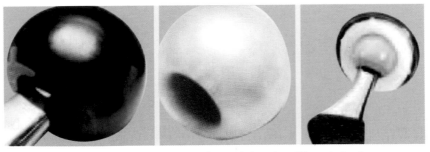

Fig. 2.11: *Ceramics*: Zirconia, alumina and zirconia reinforced alumina are various ceramic options available today

Alumina materials are brittle and much stiffer than metals. They do not tolerate impact or non-uniform loading, e.g. due to malpositioning. Fractures were reported with initial designs of ceramic heads due to improper taper fit. Zirconia has increased toughness compared to alumina. It has less stiffness and increased strength in tension compared with alumina, stainless steels, and cobalt alloys. Compressive strength of zirconia is less than alumina. Zirconia–toughened alumina formed by mixing both the materials has high strength of zirconia and thermostability of alumina.

Bone Cement

Sir John Charnley first used PMMA bone cement to anchor femoral endoprosthesis in 1958. Acrylic bone cement is a space-filling, load-transferring material, i.e. just like a grout. It does not bond chemically to bone or to the surface of metal components or UHMWPE. It is for fixation and anchoring of the prosthetic joints to the bone. In a well cemented arthroplasty of the hip there is an even load-transfer from prosthesis to the bone. Antibiotics may be added for gradual local release (Fig. 2.12).

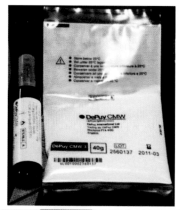

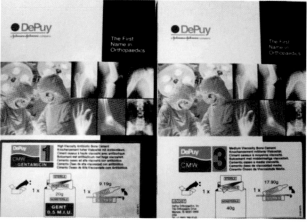

Fig. 2.12: *Bone cements*: Bone cement is available in a combination pack of a liquid and powder. These may be high viscosity or low viscosity bone cement, with or without antibiotic

Bone cement is strong in compression but weak in tension and torsion. It may undergo fatigue fracture. Particles generated by cement breakdown induce chronic inflammatory and foreign-body reaction leading to osteolysis and implant loosening the **cement disease** or more correctly the **particulate disease**.

The basic component is methylmethacrylate (MMA). It is supplied as 'two component system':
1. A monomer liquid in an ampoule and
2. A polymer powder in a pack

Liquid monomer is made up of methylmethacrylate (MMA) or butylmethacrylate, dimethyl-para-toluidine (activator), hydroquinone (stabilizer) with or without a coloring agent- Chlorophyll. **Cement powder** is a mixture of polymer powder-PMMA or MMA copolymers, diabenzoyl peroxide (initiator), $BaSO_4$/zirconium dioxide (radio-opacifier) with or without an antibiotic.

Mixing of cement powder and liquid will initially cause swelling and physical dissolution; the polymer powder takes up the monomer liquid forming viscous semisolid dough. Mixing may be done by gently stirring the mixture without entrapping air in it. Vacuum mixing is preferable. The chemical reaction follows; the initiator in the powder and the activator in the liquid produce free radicals which cause polymerization of MMA. The reaction is temperature dependent exothermic reaction. It is slower at cooler temperature. The phases of cement hardening are: mixing phase (up to 1 min), waiting phase (up to several min), working phase (2-4 min), hardening phase (1-2 min). The cement may be a high-viscosity or a low-viscosity cement depending on the waiting phase. This is dependent on the chemical composition. Do not alter powder to liquid ratio to slow down polymerization. **Pre-chilling the constituents by keeping in a refrigerator can be used to get additional working time.**

Some cemented implants are pre-coated with a thin layer of PMMA. This PMMA surface can then bind chemically to PMMA cement applied while fixing.

Articulating Surfaces in Hip Arthroplasty

The commonly used articulating surfaces are metal on polyethylene (MOP), ceramic on polyethylene (COP), ceramic on ceramic (COC) and metal on metal (MOM) and most recently ceramic on metal (COM) (Fig. 2.13):
- Materials used for MOP articulations are stainless steel (316L, F-56), Co-Cr alloy (F-75) or rarely Ti alloy (F-136) mated with UHMWPE or XLPE.
- Materials used for COP articulations are aluminia or zirconia on UHMWPE.
- Material used for MOM articulations is Co-Cr on Co-Cr alloy
- Material used for COC articulation is aluminium oxide on aluminium oxide.
- Material used for COM is zirconia toughened alumina on Co-Cr alloy.

Bearing Surfaces: MOP

Metal on polyethylene are the conventional aticulating surfaces having good initial result. However with time and usage they produce wear debris which may cause osteolysis and implant loosening.

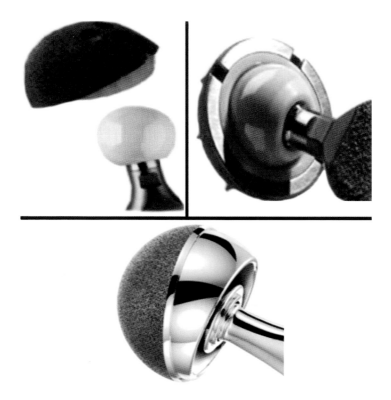

Fig. 2.13: Bearing surfaces in hip arthroplasty

Volumetric wear (*v*) is a function of radius squared ($v = r^2w$) and increases dramatically with increase in the bearing radius. An increase in bearing size from 22 mm to 32 mm doubles the volume wear for the same linear wear rate. The linear wear rate of 28 mm MOP articulation is about equal to that of 22 mm; however the volume wear of 28 mm is higher. There is no difference in wear of machined compared to compression molded PE components.

Highly Cross-linked PE (XLPE) has decreased wear rate, volume wear and lesser incidence of associated periprosthetic osteolysis. However certain doubts are being raised about its utility in arthroplasty. Sub micron wear particles released may incite greater inflammatory response. Only further clinical studies can answer if all or some of these XLPEs are favorable.

Bearing Surfaces: COP

Ceramics have relatively high hardness and abrasion resistance. These can be highly polished, have better wettability and have low coefficient of friction with PE.

Wear in some studies was however comparable to MOP. Ceramic heads are placed on a metal stems. Precise Morse taper fit is required to prevent excessive hoop stresses on ceramic head which may lead to fracture of the ceramic. Fractures reported with newer alumina are low (0.004%).

Bearing Surfaces: MOM

In 1988 second generation MOM bearings were introduced. These are carbide containing forged Co-Cr-Mo alloy. Better implant design with optimal clearance has resulted in low wear rate and anticipated longer life. These are more suitable for young patients. Large diameter bearings can be made which permit larger arc of motion with decreased impingement and associated risk of dislocation. However, there is a debate regarding its use in females of child bearing age, due to the potential teratogenicity of metal ions released in the body. Its use is contraindicated in patients with altered renal function.

Chapter Three

Relevant Anatomy and Biomechanics of the Hip

The hip joint is a ball and socket joint. The head of the femur articulates with the acetabulum (Fig. 3.1). It allows rotation and movement in coronal and sagittal planes however there can be no translation (Fig. 3.2).

The movements possible at the hip joint are flexion-extension, abduction-adduction, external and internal rotations and a combination of these circumduction.

The Proximal Femur

Femur is a long bone with multiple bows and twists. The proximal most part has an antero-medial branch out—the femoral neck with a spherical summit—the head. Lateral to this neck-shaft junction and postero-medially are bony protuberances of the greater and lesser trochanters respectively. The femoral shaft has a gentle anterior bowing. The radius of curvature of which varies from person to person, it is more in taller individuals, i.e. the curve is gentler. In the erect position the middle portion of the femur is in the coronal plane of the body and the two ends incline posteriorly to articulate with the respective joints. Besides this the proximal femur has a subtle posterior bow with the apex at the level of the lesser trochanter. The radius of this curve remains relatively constant irrespective of the length of the femur (Fig. 3.3).

The neck and the shaft make an oblique angle, the neck-shaft angle, which is variable, the average being 135°. The neck shaft angle and the neck length are the parameters that decide the horizontal and vertical femoral off-sets (Fig. 3.4). This anatomy lateralizes the insertion of hip abductors, which are attached to the greater trochanter. It improves the abductor lever arm and therefore less force is required to abduct the pelvis while walking, etc. The center of the femoral head lies at the same level as the tip of the greater trochanter, though this is not always true.

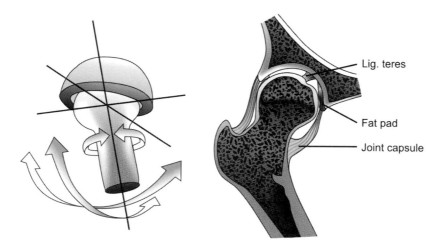

Fig. 3.1: Hip joint is a ball and socket joint with a stable bony configuration

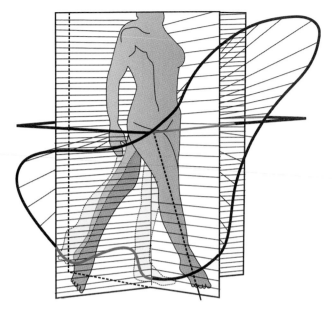

Fig. 3.2: The movements possible at the hip joint are flexion-extension, abduction-adduction, external and internal rotations and a combination of these circumduction

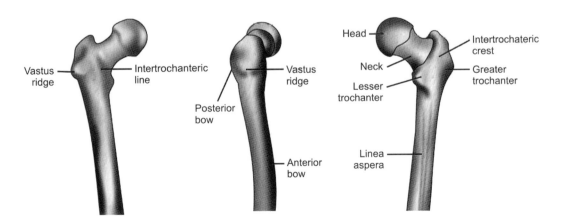

Fig. 3.3: Femur has a posterior bowing at the level of the trochanter besides the anterior bowing of the shaft

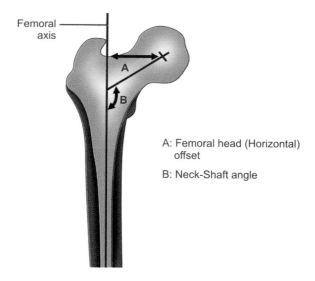

Fig. 3.4: The neck subtends an angle of about 135° to the shaft (Neck-shaft angle).
The distance of the center of the head to the femoral axis determines the femoral head (horizontal) offset

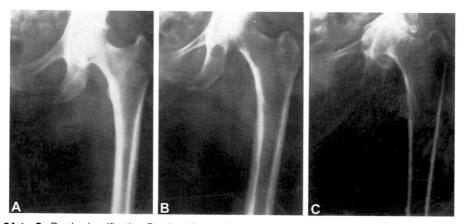

Figs. 3.5A to C: *Dorr's classification-Proximal femur.* Type A: Champagne flute, Type B: Funnel type, Type C: Stovepipe/cylindrical. Cementless femoral stems fit better into Type A and B femurs and cemented prosthesis are better suited for and type B and C femoral canals

When the femoral shaft is placed in the anatomical position, the neck and the head are directed anteriorly by about 10-15°—the femoral anteversion. This is partly due to the torsion in the proximal femur.

Dorr et al have developed a classification for proximal femoral bone quality by correlating radiographic appearance of bone and cortical index with bone mineral density. It is a widely used tool for matching femoral implant fixation in patients of total hip replacement. Dorr suggested that there are three types of proximal femur, A is the normal taper top with thick cortex, C is a clear loss of taper with thin cortex, and B is in between. Strong, dense bone with thick cortices (Dorr type A-B) are better suited for cementless fixation, whereas more osteoporotic bone (Dorr type B-C) are thought to provide the ideal substrate for optimum cement technique (Fig. 3.5).

The Acetabulum

Acetabulum on either side is formed by the fusion of three pelvic bones: ilium, ischium and pubis (Fig. 3.6). These form a bony socket which is defective antero-inferiorly. The transverse ligament of the acetabulum is a strong band of fibers that bridges this acetabular notch and is attached to its margin. It completes the rim of the acetabulum (Fig. 3.7).

The acetabular labrum is a firm fibrocartilage attached to the rim of the bony acetabulum which deepens the acetabular socket. The ligamentum teres is a ligament that attaches the femoral head to the socket.

In the erect position the anterior-superior iliac spines and the symphysis pubis lie in the coronal plane. In this position the acetabulum is directed approximately 45° laterally and 15° forward (the acetabular anteversion). The apparent anteversion increases with the flexion of the pelvis on the lumbar spine, as while sitting and in lateral decubitus position (e.g. while operating).

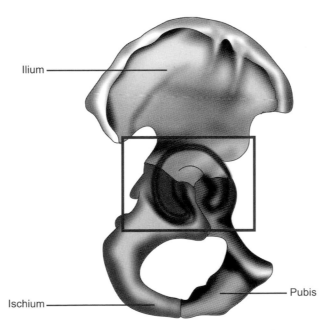

Fig. 3.6: The three pelvic bones forming the acetabular socket. In the erect position the anterior-superior iliac spines and the symphysis pubis lie in the coronal plane

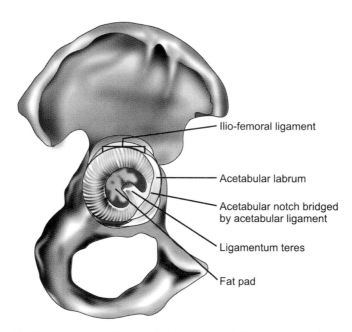

Fig. 3.7: The anatomy of the acetabular socket with the femoral head removed

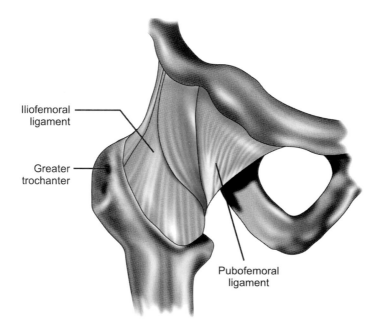

Fig. 3.8: The capsular ligaments around the hip (anterior view)—Iliofemoral and pubofemoral ligaments. Ischiofemoral ligament lies posteriorly

The capsule of the joint is proximally attached about the rim of the acetabulum and distally to the neck – anteriorly at the inter-trochanteric line and posteriorly about half an inch proximal to the inter-trochanteric crest. The capsule has three thickenings—the ligaments. Of these the Y-shaped Ilio-femoral ligament of Bigleow is the strongest. It is the chief stabilizer of the hip in the erect position (Fig. 3.8).

The Biomechanics

Of all the species only humans beside the birds have a bipedal gait. In the erect position the entire weight of the body minus that of the lower limbs is divided equally on the two femoral heads, which is about one-third the body weight on each side (Fig. 3.9). The plane of force coincides with the strongly developed trabeculae that lie in the medial portion of the femoral neck and extend upward through the superomedial aspect of the head of femur. These trabeculae are in line with the acetabular trabeculae that extend medially towards the SI joint. The trabecular pattern becomes sparser in osteoporotic proximal femur (Fig. 3.10).

In *surface replacement arthroplasty* of the hip the natural transmission of weight bearing forces is probably emulated. This is expected to have a benefical effect on the bone quality of proximal femur and acetabulum, which in turn would make subsequent revision surgery smaller and easier to perform.

The *center of gravity* of human body lies just anterior to the second sacral vertebral body. This is posterior to the axis of the joints. Thus there is a posterior bending force in the sagittal plane. The ilio-femoral ligament of Bigleow neutralizes this. This posterior deflecting forces are particularly active when trying to sit down or getup or while using the stairs or walking up an incline.

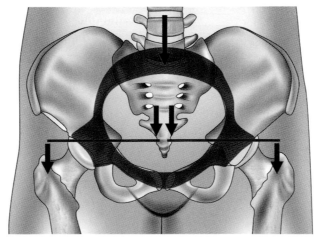

Fig. 3.9: Normally each leg bears half the body weight. The plane of force coincides with the strongly developed trabeculae that lie in the medial portion of the femoral neck and extend upward through the superomedial aspect of the head of femur. These trabeculae are in line with the acetabular trabeculae that extend medially towards the SI joint

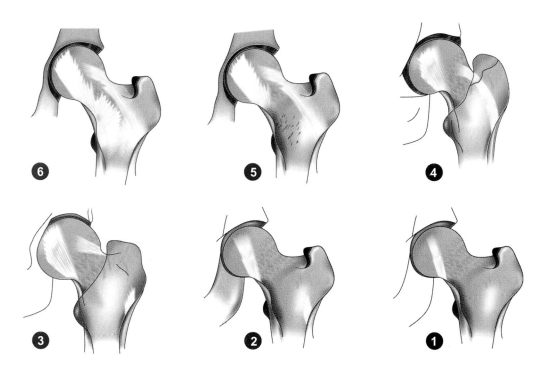

Fig. 3.10: *Singh's Index:* Pattern of trabecular resorption in the femur due to progressive osteoporosis. From 6—Normal (upper left) to 1—severe osteoporosis (lower right)

In single leg stance phase the center of gravity moves away and distal to the loaded hip. This tends to turn the body mass to the non-weight bearing side in the coronal plane. The force is counterbalanced by the combined action of abductors and other hip stabilizers viz. gluteus max, tensor fascia lata, etc. thus the pelvis tilts with the non-weight bearing side rising up. Trendelenburg sign becomes positive when this mechanism fails. Since the ratio of the length of the lever arm of the body weight with center as femoral head to the abductor lever arm is 2.5:1, the forces acting on the weight bearing femoral head is about three times the body weight. The estimated load on the femoral head during active straight leg raising is also the same (Fig. 3.11).

The mechanical axis of the lower limb passes from the center of the femoral head through the tibial spine of the knee to the center of the ankle mortice. In a normal limb a line from the center of the femoral head to the tip of the greater trochanter (Hip orientation line) is usually at about 90° to the mechanical axis. In the femur the mechanical axis runs from the center of the head to the center of the knee joint and the anatomical axis is from the piriformis fossa to the center of the knee. The two lines subtend an angle of about 6° to each other; the anatomical axis is in adduction (Fig. 3.12).

Peak contact forces across the hip joint while doing various activities have been calculated to be 5-6 times the body weight, and up to 10 times while running and jumping. Thus

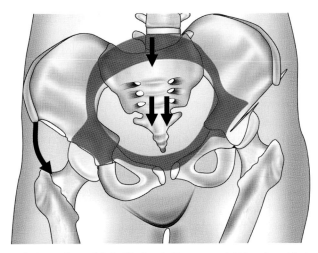

Fig. 3.11: In a single legged stance the pelvis is tilted on to the non-weight bearing side by the combined action of the opposite hip abductors. Two-thirds of the total body weight (BW) passes through the hip joint, however the net force acting is atleast 2.5 times the body weight

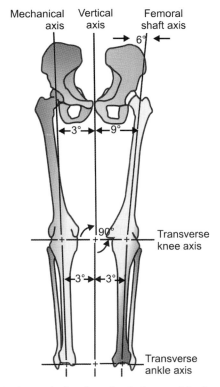

Fig. 3.12: Anatomical and mechanical axes of the lower limbs

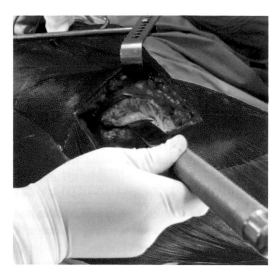

Fig. 4.3C: *Steps—anterolateral approach*: Using an osteotome a thin sliver of anterior cortex of trochanter is lifted off anteriorly

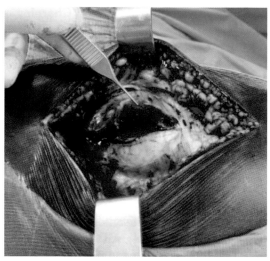

Fig. 4.3D: *Steps—anterolateral approach*: Picture after the osteotomy (Note: This is not the trochanteric osteotomy described by Charnley)

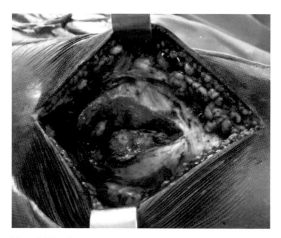

Fig. 4.3E: *Steps—anterolateral approach*: The entire extent of the incision and osteotomy now being reflected anteriorly

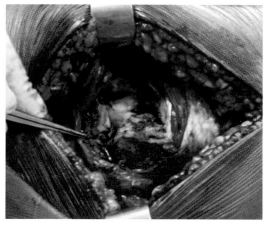

Fig. 4.3F: *Steps—anterolateral approach*: The anterior soft tissue (gluteus minimus and part of gluteus medius with the joint capsule) have been reflected anteriorly with the bone piece. Femoral neck and head is now visible

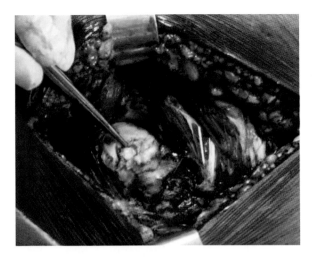

Fig. 4.3G: *Steps in anterolateral approach*: Femoral head being dislocated anteriorly here by adducting and externally rotating the hip

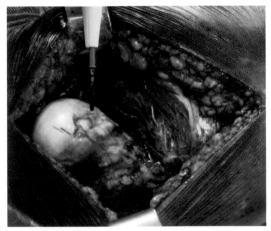

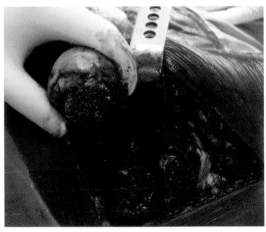

Fig. 4.3H: *Steps in anterolateral approach*: Femoral head dislocated anteriorly

Fig. 4.3I: *Steps in anterolateral approach*: Femoral neck osteotomized at a level slightly higher than the planned osteotomy

Author's Preferred Technique

We routinely perform this approach by making a lazy-S incision through gluteus medius and vastus lateralis, the *Sigma approach*. The incision is made (proximally to distally) in the tendon and distal fibres of gluteus medius through it's anterior third (along the fibers) then curving it anteriorly on the greater trochanter through the tendons of gluteus medius and minimus, then curving it posteriorly and finally along the femoral shaft through the vastus lateralis for about 5-7 cm. Proximally, the anterior fibers of the gluteus medius, the gluteus minimus and the capsule and distally the vastus lateralis are erased and reflected anteriorly as one cuff using an electro-cautery by gradually rotating the limb externally (Figs 4.4A to D). The anterior fold of tissue is then retracted forwards using the anterior hook of the Charnley retractor. This now helps to visualize the femoral neck, head and the adjacent acetabular margin (Fig. 4.4E).

The acetabular labrum is excised. Any anterior osteophyte is removed using a bone nibbler or a rongeur. Patients with an external rotation contracture may require division of the short external rotators along with the capsule (as much as possible). The femoral head is then **dislocated anteriorly** by flexing, adducting and externally rotating the thigh. The knee is held in flexion. Care is to be taken to avoid any forcible, jerky movement as this can cause a spiral fracture of the femoral shaft. The superior and inferior portions of the capsule may have to be incised as far posteriorly as possible, under direct vision. Any impinging osteophyte is removed.

If the dislocation is still not possible it is prudent to osteotomize the neck. This is done well proximal to the planned level of osteotomy, using an oscillating saw. Another cut in the proximal fragment is made parallel to this osteotomy and the intervening slice of bone removed (Figs 4.4F and G). This provides room for further manipulation. A cork-screw is then introduced into the femoral head which is then levered out of the socket (Figs 4.4H and I). Thickened ligamentum teres, if present, may have to be incised with a sharp knife or diathermy. If dislocation of the head is still not possible, the bone is removed piece-meal after carefully fragmenting it with a chisel.

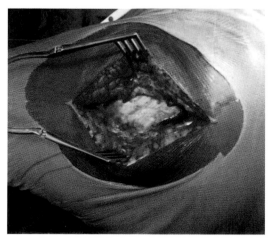 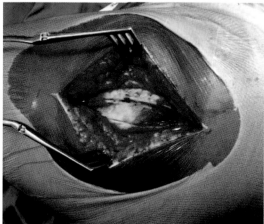

Fig. 4.4A: *Sigma approach–surgical steps:* Direct lateral incision (*Note:* the head end is at the right side of the picture)

Fig. 4.4B: *Sigma approach–surgical steps:* Iliotibial band incised along the skin incision

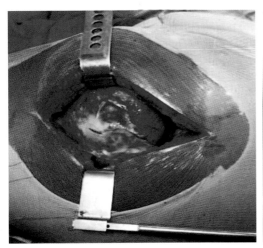

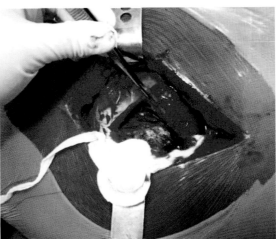

Fig. 4.4C: *Sigma approach—surgical steps*: Trochanter exposed. A lazy-S incision at the insertion of anterior fibers of gluteus medius and minimus on the anterior aspect of trochanter

Fig. 4.4D: *Sigma approach—surgical steps*: Incision on the trochanter deepened anteriorly along the neck of femur at the same time externally rotating the limb

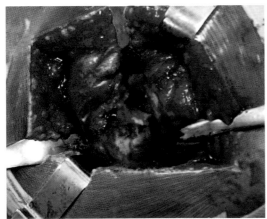

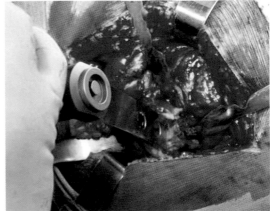

Fig. 4.4E: *Sigma approach—surgical steps*: Picture taken while looking at the operative wound from the head end : fracture neck of femur appreciated. In other hip pathologies the hip is dislocated first and then the neck osteotomized

Fig. 4.4F: *Sigma approach—surgical steps*: Femoral neck being osteotomized at the desired level to improve subsequent visibility of the acetabulum

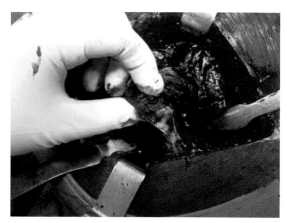
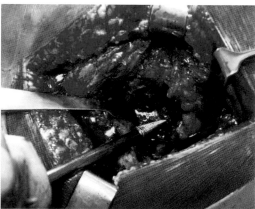

Fig. 4.4G: *Sigma approach—surgical steps*: A sliver of bone removed, base of the neck preserved

Fig. 4.4H: *Sigma approach—surgical steps*: Femoral head is now being extracted out using a myomectomy screw

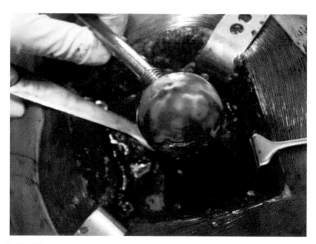

Fig. 4.4I: *Sigma approach—surgical steps*: Femoral head seen here after removal from acetabulum (Acetabular bed seen in the background)

Exposure of Acetabulum

After dislocation of the hip, the proximal femur is delivered into the wound with a broad, flat retractor. The femoral neck is then osteotomized with an oscillating or reciprocating power saw (Figs 4.4G to I). The level of osteotomy is kept a few mm proximal to the intended femoral neck osteotomy. The femoral head is removed from the wound. Any soft tissue attachment is removed. The cancellous bone from the head extracted may be used as a source of graft, if need be. The acetabulum is exposed by retracting the femur posteriorly

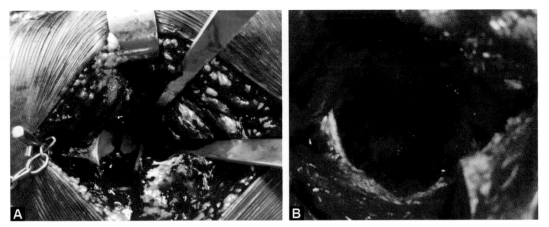

Figs 4.5A and B: *Acetabular exposure antero-lateral approach:* (A) Acetabulum is exposed after osteotomy of the neck and removal of femoral head. The three retractors are placed superiorly (a pin retractor), antero-inferiorly into the obturator foramen and postero-inferiorly over the body of the ischium (two Hohmann's retractors), (B) Acetabular bed after reaming. Note the oozing cancellous bone

and inferiorly using a Hohmann's retractor on the ischium posteriorly. A second short tipped retractor is placed anterosuperiorly between the anterior lip of the acetabulum and the psoas tendon (10 and 2 O'clock for left and right hip respectively). Pin retractors may be used alternatively. A third broad retractor is placed beneath the transverse acetabular ligament to provide exposure inferiorly (Fig. 4.5A). The acetabulum is prepared by incremental reaming (Fig. 4.5B).

TOTAL HIP ARTHROPLASTY THROUGH POSTEROLATERAL APPROACH, WITH POSTERIOR DISLOCATION OF HIP

Posterolateral approach is a modification of posterior approaches described by Gibson and by Moore. It can be extended distally to approach the entire femoral shaft, if need be. It is a popular approach for both primary and revision total hip arthroplasty.

The patient is firmly anchored in the straight lateral position with the side to be operated upon facing the ceiling. A slightly curved skin incision is made centered over the greater trochanter, starting proximally at a point about the level of the anterosuperior iliac spine along a line parallel to the posterior edge of the greater trochanter (Fig. 4.6A). The incision is extended distally to the center of the greater trochanter and then along the course of the femoral shaft to a point 8-10 cm distally. The subcutaneous tissue is divided along the skin incision in a single plane down to the fascia lata and the thin fascia covering the gluteus maximus superiorly. The incision is deepened to divide the fascia in line with the skin wound. Gluteus maximus is split proximally by blunt dissection in the direction of the fibers maintaining hemostasis and distally far enough to expose the tendinous insertion of the gluteus maximus on the femoral shaft posteriorly (Fig. 4.6B).

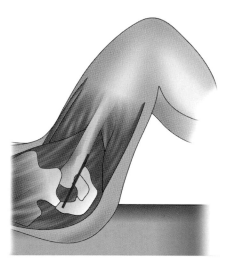

Fig. 4.6A: *Posterolateral approach*: The incision is centered over the posterior aspect of the greater trochanter with a gentle backward slope proximally

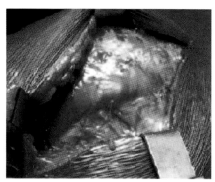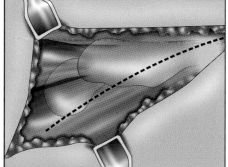

Fig. 4.6B: *Posterolateral approach*: Exposure following incision of skin, deep fascia and gluteus maximus (retracted with Charnley retractor)

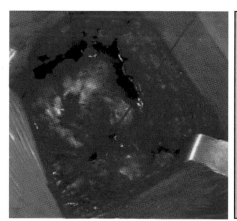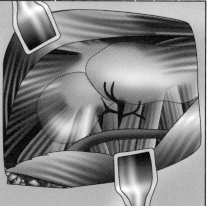

Fig. 4.6C: *Posterolateral approach*: Short external rotators exposed and marked here are then erased after tagging with tie suture carefully protecting the sciatic nerve along with it

Charnley's retractor is placed beneath the fascia lata at the level of the trochanter. The trochanteric bursa is divided and erased posteriorly to expose the short external rotators and the posterior edge of the gluteus medius. With the hip in extension and the knee flexed the femur is internally rotated to make the short external rotators taut and visible. The sciatic nerve is palpated with a finger as it passes superficial to the obturator internus and the gemelli (complete exposure of the nerve is usually not required) (Fig. 4.6C).

The tendinous insertions of the piriformis and obturator internus are palpated and tagged with sutures for later identification at closure. The short external rotators are divided, including at least the proximal half of the quadratus femoris, close to the insertion on the femur. Hemostasis is achieved (blood vessels are located along the piriformis tendon). The short external rotators are reflected posteriorly, protecting the sciatic nerve. The interval between the gluteus medius and the superior capsule is dissected and Hohmann's retractors are inserted superiorly and inferiorly to obtain exposure of the entire superior, posterior, and inferior portions of the capsule. The exposed portion of the capsule is divided along its attachment on the femur. The visible portion of the capsule may be excised, or preferably retracted. The acetabular labrum is excised.

The hip is dislocated posteriorly by flexing, adducting, and gently internally rotating the hip (Fig. 4.6D). A bone hook may be placed beneath the femoral neck at the level of the lesser trochanter to gently lift the head out of the acetabulum, if required. The ligamentum teres which usually avulses during dislocation may sometimes require division before the femoral head can be delivered out. No forcible movement is to be attempted as this can cause a spiral fracture of the shaft. Ensure the release of superior and inferior portions of the capsule as far anteriorly as possible, if need be. Any osteophyte along the posterior rim

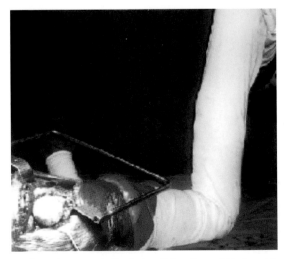

Fig. 4.6D: *Posterolateral approach*: Posterior dislocation of hip is achieved by flexing, internally rotating and adducting the hip joint

of the acetabulum is removed. If the hip still cannot be dislocated, the femoral neck is osteotomized with an oscillating saw at a level just proximal to the planned osteotomy and the head removed with a corkscrew or if required the head is removed piece-meal.

After dislocation of the hip, the proximal femur is delivered into the wound with a broad, flat retractor. The femoral neck is then osteotomized with an oscillating or reciprocating power saw. The level of cut is about 2 mm proximal to the intended femoral neck osteotomy. The extracted head may be used as a source of bone graft, if need be. Prior to dislocating the hip a pin may be inserted into the ilium superiorly and then a mark made at a fixed point on the greater trochanter, the distance measured. The same is used to assess limb length status post-operatively.

Exposure of Acetabulum

The femur is retracted anteriorly with a bone hook and the capsule is placed under tension (Fig. 4.6E). The anterior capsule is divided and a curved sharp tipped Hohmann's retractor is placed strictly in the interval between the anterior lip of the acetabulum and the psoas tendon (10 and 2 O'clock for left and right hip respectively). Injury to the femoral nerve and vessels is carefully avoided. A broad retractor is placed beneath the transverse acetabular ligament to provide inferior exposure. The posterior soft tissues are retracted with a right-angle retractor placed on top of a laparotomy sponge (to avoid compression or excessive traction on the sciatic nerve). As an alternative, pin retractor may be placed into the posterior column or a sharp Hohmann's retractor may be inserted just superior to the ischium for

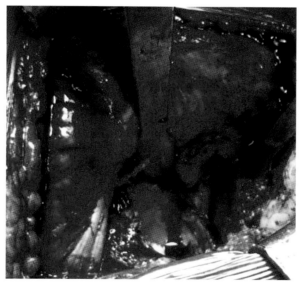

Fig. 4.6E: *Posterolateral approach*: Acetabular exposure through the posterior approach

soft tissue retraction. Care is to be taken to avoid injury to the sciatic nerve or placing the pins within the acetabulum where they will interfere with acetabular preparation. The femur is then retracted anteriorly and medially and rotated to the best position for acetabular exposure. Very rarely, if the exposure is still not adequate the tendinous insertion of the gluteus maximus on femur is divided (a 1-cm stump of tendon is left for ease of reattachment).

Preparation of Acetabulum and Femur

The preparation of the acetabulum and the femoral medullary canal in principle is similar for both the cementless and the cemented total hip arthroplasty.

Preparation of Acetabulum

Once the acetabulum is exposed using either of the approaches, the labrum and remaining capsule is excised. The knife blade should be within the confines of the acetabulum at all times to avoid injury to important structures both anteriorly and posteriorly. The bony margins of the rim of the acetabulum are exposed around its entire circumference to facilitate proper visualization and placement of the acetabular component. Osteotome or nibbler is used to remove osteophytes that protrude beyond the bony limits of the true acetabulum.

Once the acetabulum is well exposed the ligamentum teres stump is excised and remaining soft tissue curetted out from the region of the pulvinar. Any bleeder if encountered is cauterized. Transverse acetabular ligament if hypertrophic is excised to accommodate the correct sized reamers in the acetabulum.

Hypertrophic osteophytes at the floor of the acetabulum can be palpated and have to be removed with nibblers and rongeurs. Large osteophytes prevent proper assessment of the true location of the medial wall leading to lateralized placement of the acetabular component. In such a situation medially directed reaming is done first, using a small sized acetabular reamer. This will not only allow correct medio-lateral placement but also improve lateral coverage of the component. Avoid over reaming or damaging the medial wall.

The subsequent reamers are directed in the same plane as the opening face of the acetabulum keeping the femur retracted (Figs 4.6E and F). If the femur is not adequately retracted away, it may misdirect the reamers posteriorly or anteriorly, depending on the approach used and may cause eccentric reaming of the acetabular wall. Progressively larger reamers in 1- or 2-mm increments are used. The acetabulum is assessed regularly for the depth of reaming. Reaming is complete when all cartilage has been removed, the reamers have cut bone out to the periphery of the acetabulum, a hemispherical shape has been produced and a bleeding subchondral bone-bed is exposed. Any remaining soft tissue, subchondral cyst from the floor of the acetabulum is curetted and any overhanging soft tissue around the periphery of the acetabulum is excised. The cavity is filled with morselized cancellous bone obtained from the patient's femoral head. The graft is impacted with a small hemi-spherical bone punch.

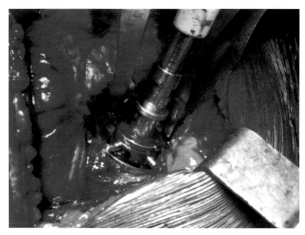

Fig. 4.6F: *Posterolateral approach:* Acetabular bed being reamed

The true lateral position is ensured before insertion of the acetabular component. Proceed with implantation of a cementless or cemented acetabular component.

Adequate extension of the upper portion of the incision may be required for reaming of the femoral canal from a superior direction, and the distal extension of the exposure for preparation and insertion of the acetabular component from an antero-inferior direction.

Femoral Neck Osteotomy and Preparation for Femoral Stem

A wide retractor is placed under the greater trochanter to aid in lifting the proximal femur. The leg is then pulled in maximal flexion and adduction and external rotation for anteriorly dislocated or internal rotation for posteriorly dislocated hip. The adjacent soft tissue especially the abductors are protected with the retractors. Preparation of femoral stem involves:

a. Neck osteotomy
b. Entry point for femoral reaming
c. Femoral reaming and
d. Femoral broaching.

The neck is osteotomized at the appropriate level after palpating the lesser trochanter. The proximal end of the neck is visualized properly by adjusting the position of the thigh. The cancellous bone is gouged out from the center of exposed bone at the base of the neck of femur. The femoral canal is then explored with a long curette to determine the direction of reaming. The canal is then prepared by using the hip system chosen. Be careful to insert the reamers and the broaches as laterally as possible to avoid the complications of medial perforation and varus placement of the prosthetic stem (See Chapter 7 and 8 for detailed steps of surgery).

The patients planned for hemiarthroplasty the femoral head size is measured and the prosthetic size chosen accordingly.

Chapter Five

Indications and Contraindications for Total Hip Arthroplasty

The foremost in Total hip replacement is choosing the right prosthesis for the right diagnosis. Therefore it is important to assess the patient for the right indication. The planning and treatment is done accordingly. This is achieved by a thorough *clinico-radiological examination* to ascertain the cause of pain/disability (Fig. 5.1).

Clinico-radiological Examination: To Ascertain the Cause of Pain and Disability

Localization of site of pain and pathology is necessary before one embarks upon any treatment for the patient. Pain in the groin is more specific for hip disease.

*   Spine pathology should be ruled out. Co-existing hip and spine pathologies are known.

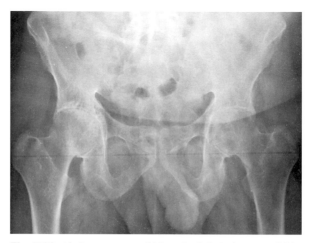

Fig. 5.1A: *Various causes of hip pain*: Ankylosing spondylitis

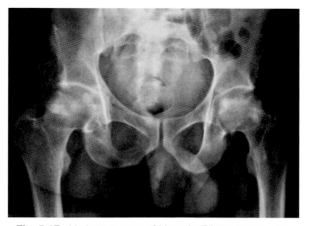

Fig. 5.1B: *Various causes of hip pain*: Bilateral avascular necrosis hip

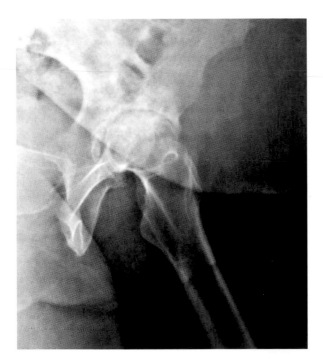

Fig. 5.1C: *Various causes of hip pain*: Rheumatoid arthritis

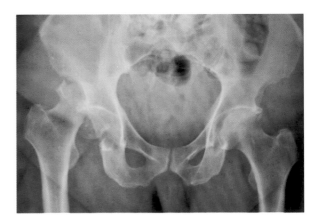

Fig. 5.1D: *Various causes of hip pain*: Neglected fracture dislocation right hip

- Intra-pelvic pathologies may present with groin pain. The differential diagnosis includes inguinal hernia, retro-cecal appendix, ovarian cyst.
- Hip pain may be referred to the knee and vice-versa; and one needs to be careful.
- Extra-articular causes of hip pain are trochanteric/psoas bursitis, abductor/adductor strain, ischio-gluteal bursitis, etc.

On physical examination pain and limitation of hip rotation, pain on hip loading or a positive Stinchfield test (pain on resisted hip flexion) is suggestive of intra-articular hip pathology as the cause of pain.

Once intra-articular hip pathology has been established as the cause of pain, establish the diagnosis. This would decide the future course of treatment. Avascular necrosis (AVN) of hip, inflammatory arthritis, infection, metastatic disease, trauma and dysplasia are the common causes. Different etio-pathologies need to be handled differently, as the disease process may have different extent of involvement. Inflammatory pathologies may have multi-system and poly-articular involvement. These patients may be on disease modifying drugs and/or steroids which need to be altered/ stopped if hip replacement or any other surgical procedure is being planned. Acute flare up of gout needs to be corrected before any surgical intervention. Sickle cell anemia a cause of AVN also alters hematological parameters which may need to be addressed. AVN usually also involves the other hip which if anatomically preserved can be considered for head preserving surgery. Hip replacement is contraindicated in active infective pathologies.

Trial of Alternative Treatment Options

Conservative measures including weight loss, anti-inflammatory medication, reasonable modification of activity, and use of a cane should be advised. Often these measures relieve the symptoms enough to make surgery unnecessary or at least delay the need for surgery for a significant period. In a young individual with a physically demanding occupation, consideration should be given to change to a more sedentary vocation. If the demand on the hip is lessened, the need for surgery may be delayed.

Non-arthroplasty interventions described are pelvic and femoral osteotomy. Arthroscopy of the hip is described for patients with labral tear or loose body. Resection arthroplasty and arthodesis are certain treatment options available which may not be very acceptable to the patient but are still valuable in extreme cases. Core decompression with or without vascularized bone graft are treatment options for early AVN of femoral head.

Indications for Total Hip Arthroplasty

The main objectives of total hip arthroplasty are, in order of priority: relief of pain, stability, mobility, and equal leg length. The primary indication for total hip arthroplasty is alleviation of incapacitating pain followed by improved function of the hip (Fig. 5.2).

The current list of indications is:
- Arthritis
  - Rheumatoid arthritis
  - Degenerative joint disease
    - Primary
    - Secondary (to intra-articular fractures of the hip joint , dislocation hip, dysplasia of hip, avascular necrosis of femoral head, Perthes disease, Paget's disease) (Fig. 5.3).
  - Sequlae of infective arthritis (pyogenic/ tubercular)

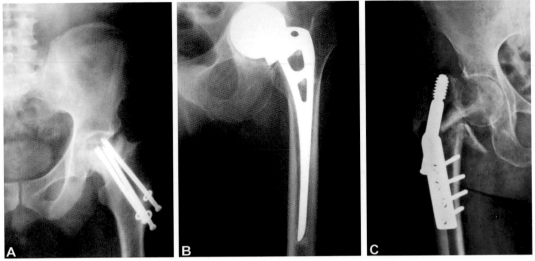

Figs 5.2A to C: *Failed reconstruction hip*: (A) Failed osteosynthesis—fracture neck of femur with AVN of femoral head, (B) Painful hip following hemiarthroplasty (Austin-Moore prosthesis), (C) Failed DHS

- Non-union femoral neck or trochanteric fractures
- Displaced femoral neck and trochanteric fracture in the elderly patients
- Congenital dislocation hip
- Hip fusion/arthrodesis
- Failed reconstruction
- Bony tumor involving proximal femur and acetabulum.

Patients over 60 years of age were considered the most suitable candidates for total hip arthroplasty. Many older individuals of 80 years or more are now undergoing total hip arthroplasty successfully. Poor outcomes appear to be related more to co-morbidities than to age alone.

'THR is an option for nearly all patients with diseases of the hip that cause chronic discomfort and significant functional impairment.' However, in younger individuals, total hip arthroplasty is not the only reconstruction procedure available for a painful hip. Procedures like arthrodesis and osteotomies are good options. Core decompression, vascularized fibular grafting, and osteotomy should be considered for patients with avascular necrosis of the femoral head, especially when involvement is limited. The potential for loosening and osteolysis and requirement of repeated revision surgeries is more in young patients after total hip arthroplasty. However the scene is gradually changing with the advent of newer designs and surfaces of implants which provide longevity to the procedure with an added ability to pursue near normal life-style. At the same time these do not make revision surgeries complicated.

However delaying a replacement has a distinct advantage of possible improvement in the techniques and implants during this period.

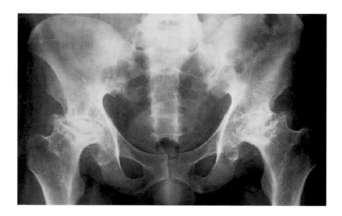

Fig. 5.3: *AVN*: Bilateral AVN hip with secondary OA

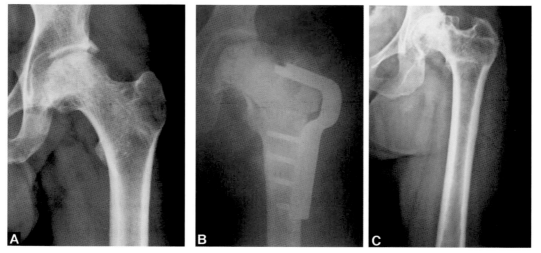

Figs 5.4A to C: *AVN femoral head*: (A) After core decompression, (B) Following corrective osteotomy (C) Now with painful hip; late secondary OA after hardware removal

Surgery is justified if despite conservative measures, pain at night and pain with motion and weight-bearing is severe enough to prevent the patient from working or from carrying out the activities of daily living. Pain in the presence of a destructive process in the hip joint as evidenced on radiographs is also an indication for surgery (Fig. 5.4).

Contraindications for Total Hip Arthroplasty

Total hip arthroplasty is a major surgical procedure associated with a significant number of complications and probable mortality. Patients must hence be evaluated carefully, especially for systemic disorders and for general debility that may contraindicate an elective major operation. Preoperative medical consultation is recommended as it may pick up unsuspected problems requiring correction before hip surgery.

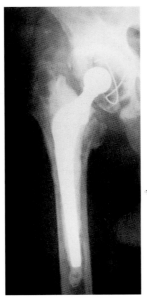

Fig. 5.5: *Infected hip*: Note radiolucency around the trochanter

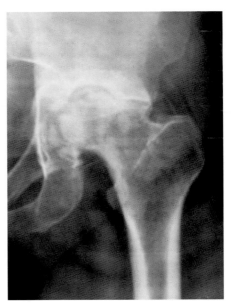

Fig. 5.6: Secondary OA following fracture dislocation hip: AVN with collapsed femoral head with deformed acetabulum

Specific, absolute contraindications for total hip arthroplasty include:
- Active infection of the hip joint or any other region and (Fig. 5.5)
- Any unstable medical illnesses that would significantly increase the risk of morbidity or mortality.

Relative contraindications include:
- Any process that is rapidly destroying bone,
- Neuropathic arthropathy,
- An absence or relative insufficiency of the abductor musculature, and
- Rapidly progressive neurological diseases.

Patients with limitation of motion, limp, or leg length inequality but with little or no hip pain are not candidates for total hip arthroplasty.

Decision making in arthroplasty is as important today as it was ever. It is a permanent change in the patient's body. One should realize as Harkess writes in Campbell's Orthopedics, 'There is no doubt that the primary total hip arthroplasty offers the best chance of success. Therefore the selection of the appropriate patient, the proper implants and the technical performance of the operation are of utmost importance (Fig. 5.6).'

Chapter Six

Total Hip Arthroplasty—
Planning

Hip replacement has evolved significantly in the past two decades. Primary THA, currently, has various options of the components that may be used to recreate the cup of the acetabulum and femoral head and neck (with the stem). It may be a conventional hip replacement or a surface replacement where indicated. The prosthetic acetabulum may be cemented or cementless press-fit socket. The cementless cup may be a monobloc metal implant or may have a liner. The liner may be made up of polyethylene, metal, polyethylene backed metal or a ceramic. The femoral stems, again, may be cemented or cementless. The cemented may be with a regular finish or a polished taper finish. The cementless stem may be fabricated of cobalt chromium, titanium or composites. These may be extensively porous coated stem or may be the proximal in-growth stem. The surface treatment may include sintered beads, plasma spray, titanium fiber metal and corundmization with or without HA coating. The femoral head and neck may be a part of the monobloc stem but now, more commonly, these are modular components. Thus the femoral neck length may be fine tuned to get a snug fit stable hip. The femoral head size may be as large as the normal contralateral hip to 32 mm to 28 mm to 22.225 mm sized Charnley's hip. The modular head may be metal or ceramic. Most surgeons agree that cemented femoral stem fixation is not appropriate in heavy young, active patients especially if the bone stock is good. Callaghan et al (Master's Technique in Orthopedic Surgery- The Hip, 2nd edition.) recommend cemented stem in patients over 65 to 70 years old, sedentary and weight less than 175 pounds.

The implant selection would be determined by the following factors:
- Age
- Weight
- Activity level
- Patient requirement
- Budget.

PLANNING TOTAL HIP ARTHROPLASTY

The key to achieve optimal result after a THA lies in meticulous pre-operative planning. This prepares the surgeon to anticipate and prepare for the possible complications. The foremost in this is choosing the right surgery for the right diagnosis. The planning of THA thus includes:

Clinico-radiological examination: to ascertain the cause of pain/disability.

Trial of alternative treatment options, if possible.

Patient assessment: to determine surgical fitness

Physical examination: relevant to THA.

Standard radiographs examination for THA planning.

Templating: to assess optimum implant; its size and placement.

Once intra-articular hip pathology has been established as the cause of pain and the diagnosis ascertained; the patient is worked up for surgery. A trial of conservative management or non-arthroplasty procedures should always be contemplated prior to attempting total hip replacement.

Patient Assessment: To Determine Surgical Fitness

Hip joint replacement is an irreversible procedure with inherent risks like infection and dislocation. The patient should realize that after a conventional arthroplasty he/she will have to forego ground level activity. With this in mind and after a fair trial of conservative management if the patient is still wanting improvement in quality of life then he/she needs to undergo hip joint replacement surgery. The patients especially the elderlies need to be evaluated for medical ailments (such as diabetes, hypertension, urinary tract/cardiac/lung ailment) and assessed for body reserve to undergo the procedure without any threat to life. Also, there should be a desire on the part of the patient to participate in the process of healing. Such patients recover earlier and stronger.

Skin at the site of incision should be healthy. Any potential source of infection should be eliminated prior to joint replacement, particularly that of skin, dental and of urinary tract.

Pre-operative mobility status and activity level determines the post-operative rehabilitation.

Physical Examination: Relevant to THA

- Local skin condition
- Previous operative scar
- Any boil or toe nail infection
- Distal neurovascular status
- Muscle strength around the hip and upper limbs
- Limb-length discrepancy using block test
- Fixed pelvic obliquity
- Exaggerated lumbar lordosis, such patients have altered acetabular orientation in erect position
- Fixed deformities at the hip, including rotational deformities
- Active and passive range of motion at the hip.
- Status of other joints (Hip replacement is usually performed prior to ipsilateral knee replacement, if required).

HIP SCORING

The assessment of hip condition and functioning prior to surgery and the response to total hip replacement is becoming a common practice. These are based on patient function and satisfaction. Various systems of assessment are available to objectively ascertain the functioning of hip. These assess the pain, the functional ability, patient satisfaction and the radiological results. The commonly used systems are
- Harris Hip evaluation score
- Oxford Hip score
- UCLA Hip score

Harris Hip Evaluation Score (Table 6.1)

Table 6.1: Harris hip evaluation score is good preoperative and postoperative tool

Patient name: _____ Age: _____ Sex: _____

Reg. no.: _____DOA: _____ Date of operation: _____

Pain

None or ignores it (44)

Slight, occasional, no compromise in activities (40)

Mild pain, no effect on average activities, rarely moderate pain with unusual activity, may take aspirin (30)

Moderate pain, tolerable but makes concessions to pain, some limitation of ordinary activity or work, may require occasional pain medicine stronger than aspirin (20)

Marked pain, serious limitation of activities (10)

Totally disabled, crippled, pain in bed, bedridden (10)

Limp

None (11)

Moderate (5)

Slight (8)

Severe (0)

Support

None (11)

Cane for long walks (7)

Cane most of the time (5)

One crutch (3)

Two canes (2)

Two crutches (0)

Note able to walk (0)

Distance walked

Unlimited (11)

Six blocks (8)

Two or three blocks (5)

Indoors only (2)

Bed and chair (0)

Stairs

Normally without using a railing (4)

Normally using a railing (2)

In any manner (1)

Unable to do stairs (0)

Table 6.1 contd...

Put on shoes and socks

With ease (4)

With difficulty (2)

Unable (0)

Sitting

Comfortably in ordinary chair one hour (5)

On a high chair for one-half hour (3)

Unable to sit comfortably in any chair (0)

Enter public transportation (1)

Yes   No

Flexion contracture: _____ **(degrees)**

Leg length discrepancy: _____ **(cm)**

Absence of deformity (all yes = 4, less than 4 = 0)

Less than 30° fixed flexion contracture

Yes   No

Less than 10° fixed adduction

Yes   No

Less than 10° fixed internal rotation in extension

Yes   No

Limb length discrepancy less than 3.2 cm

Yes   No

Range of motion (*normal)

Total degree measurements, then check range to obtain score

Flexion (*140°)

Abduction (*40°)

Adduction (*40°)

Internal rotation (*40°)

External rotation (*40°)

Range of motion scale

211°-300° (5)

161°-210° (4)

101°-160° (3)

61°-100° (2)

31°-60° (1)

0-30° (0)

Range of motion score: _____

Total Harris hip score: _____

The Harris hip score is a scale from 1-100 that assesses patient's level of pain and function. The highest possible score of 100 indicates pain free normal functional ability. The lowest possible score of 0 indicates severe pain and handicap. The factors assessed are

- Pain (max. score 44; min.0)
- Limp (max. score 11; min.0)
- Support used, if any (max. score 11; min.0)
- Distance walked (max. score 11; min.0)
- Stair usage (max. score 4; min.0)
- Ability to put on shoes and socks (max. score 4; min.0)
- Ability to sit up and its duration (max. score 5; min.0)
- Ability to use public transport (max. score 1; min.0)

The other two points assessed are on physical examination by the clinician based on:

- The presence or absence of fixed deformities; limb length discrepancy and
- Range of motion assessment.

The score of 90-100 is excellent, 80-89 being good, 70-79 fair, 60 –69 poor and below 60 a failed result.

A preoperative and a subsequent post-operative evaluation give an objective assessment of the gain to the patient. The HHS results also allow a comparative assessment of hip replacement functioning larger group of patients.

There are individual variables unrelated to the hip joint which may adversely affect the hip score, e.g. a patient with respiratory compromise unable to walk enough distance.

Oxford Hip Score (Table 6.2)

The Oxford hip score (OHS) is a joint specific outcome measure tool designed to assess disability in patients undergoing total hip replacement. The OHS is a patient–centered questionnaire that is designed to assess the functional ability and pain from the patient's perspective.

It is a twelve item questionnaire to be completed by the patient. It correlates well with patient satisfaction. It is calculated on the basis of the score of the 12 questions on activities of daily living.

For each question the respondent chooses one of the five alternative answers. The normal function score is 1, and with increasing disability the score increases to a maximum of 5. The minimum total score possible is 12, i.e. normal function and the maximum is 60, i.e. the most severe disability.

UCLA Hip Score

University of California Los Angeles (UCLA) score determines the activity level of the patient. It is rated from 1 to 10; 1 being the lowest, the patient completely dependent on others, at 10 the patient is regularly participating in impact sports.

Table 6.2: Oxford hip score is a patient centric evaluation system

1. During the past 4 weeks, how would you describe the pain you usually had from your hip?

None[1]	Very mild[2]	Mild[3]	Moderate[4]	Severe[5]

2. During the past 4 weeks, have you had any trouble with washing and drying yourself (all over) because of your hip?

No trouble at all[1]	Very little trouble[2]	Moderate trouble[3]	Extreme difficulty[4]	Impossible to do[5]

3. During the past 4 weeks, have you had any trouble getting in and out of a car or using public transport because of your hip?

No trouble at all[1]	Very little trouble[2]	Moderate trouble[3]	Extreme difficulty[4]	Impossible to do[5]

4. During the past 4 weeks, have you been able to put on a pair of socks, stocking or tights?

Yes, easily[1]	With little difficulty[2]	With moderate difficulty[3]	With extreme difficulty[4]	No, impossible[5]

5. During the past 4 weeks, could you do the household shopping on your own?

Yes, easily[1]	With little difficulty[2]	With moderate difficulty[3]	With extreme difficulty[4]	No, impossible[5]

6. During the past 4 weeks for how long have you been able to walk before pain from your hip becomes severe (with or without a stick)?

No pain/more than 30 minutes[1]	16-30 minutes[2]	5-15 minutes[3]	Around the house only[4]	Not at all-pain severe on walking[5]

7. During the past 4 weeks, have you been able to climb a flight of stairs?

Yes, easily[1]	With little difficulty[2]	With moderate difficulty[3]	With extreme difficulty[4]	No, impossible[5]

8. During the past 4 weeks, after a meal (sat at a table), how painful has it been for you to stand up from a chair because of your hip?

Not at all painful[1]	Slightly painful[2]	Moderately Painful[3]	Very painful[4]	Unbearable[5]

9. During the past 4 weeks, have you been limping when walking because of your hip?

Rarely/never[1]	Sometimes, or just at first[2]	Often, not just at first[3]	Most of the time[4]	All of the time[5]

10. During the past 4 weeks, have you had any sudden or severe pain-'shooting', 'stabbing' or 'spasms'- from the affected hip?

No days[1]	Only 1 or 2 days[2]	Some days[3]	Most days[4]	Every day[5]

11. During the past 4 weeks, how much pain from your hip has interfered with your usual work (including housework)?

Not at all[1]	A little bit[2]	Moderately[3]	Greatly[4]	Totally[5]

12. During the past 4 weeks, have you been troubled by pain from your hip in bed at night?

No night[1]	Only 1 or 2 nights[2]	Some nights[3]	Most nights[4]	Every night[5]

TEMPLATING

Restoring normal hip biomechanics is the objective of total hip replacement. Templating prepares the surgeon in achieving this goal. The target is to restore:
- Anatomic center of rotation of the hip joint
- Femoral offset (Horizontal offset)
- Vertical offset (Fig. 6.1)

Horizontal offset is the distance between center of rotation of head and the axis of femoral shaft. It determines abductor moment arm.

Vertical offset is the distance between center of head (rotation) and lesser trochanter.

Tear drop radiological mark depicting infero-medial limit of acetabulum. It determines leg length. Resotration of limb length and abduction moment arm restores biomechanics of the hip joint.

Templating helps in:
- Deciding the implant (cemented, cementless etc.)
- Size of the implant required
- Predicting the need for special instruments, e.g. bone grafting/wiring/fixation sets.

Standard Radiographs Examination for THA Planning

Radiographs taken are:
- *Pelvis with both hips*: AP view (with upper half of thigh) [Fig. 6.2A]
- *Affected hip*: AP view in ~ 20^0 of internal rotation (unless hip movements restricted).
- *Affected hip*: Lateral view (with upper half of thigh) [Fig. 6.2B].

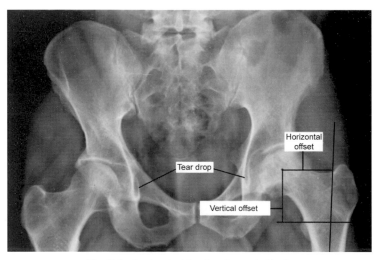

Fig. 6.1: Anatomical landmarks and offsets

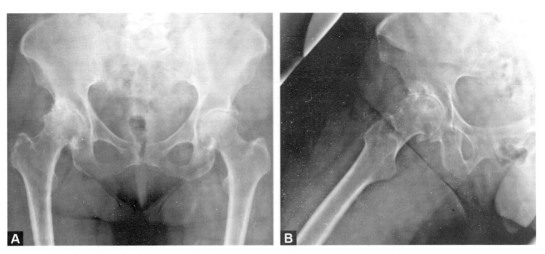

Fig. 6.2: *Standard X-ray: pelvis with both hips*: (A) X-ray pelvis with both hips with upper half thighs anteroposterior view, (B) X-ray right hip with thigh lateral view

MEASUREMENTS ON ANTEROPOSTERIOR RADIOGRAPH OF PELVIS WITH HIPS

Determining Limb Length Discrepancy

Draw inter tear-drop line. Next draw a line connecting identical points on the lesser trochanter (Fig. 6.3). Any difference on the two sides is the true difference in the limb lengths of either side.

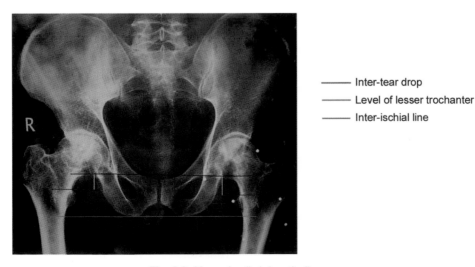

———— Inter-tear drop
———— Level of lesser trochanter
———— Inter-ischial line

Fig. 6.3: Measuring limb-length discrepancy

Acetabular Templating

Acetabular templating is done by placing the template of the cup which is of the appropriate size, extending from the supero-lateral margin of the acetabulum up to the lateral margin of the tear drop inferomedially. The inferior margin is at the proximal level of obturator foramen. Mark the center of the acetabular component on the radiograph. This is the center of rotation of the hip joint. The horizontal and vertical distance from the tear drop to the templated center of rotation is checked. This is compared to the values on the unaffected side. Make an index mark superior to the center of rotation if the side to be operated upon is short depending upon the limb length discrepancy. This is relevant particularly if the shortening is on the acetabular side. Correction of up to 3 cm length is a reasonable target.

There should be a minimal need of removal of sub-chondral bone. In a cemented cup arthroplasty an additional gap of 2-3 mm should be left for the thickness of cement mantle all around the cup (Fig. 6.4).

In patients with protrusio acetabuli the center of rotation needs to be lateralized. Since the central defect needs to be grafted the purchase of the component is achieved using an oversized acetabulum with a peripheral rim contact. The disadvantages of not correcting protrusion (medialized acetabulum) include; shortening, impingement, of neck on the cup and poor abductor mechanism.

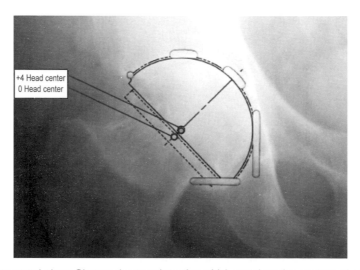

Fig. 6.4: Templating acetabulum: Choose the template size which matches the contour of acetabulum without removal of excessive subchondral bone. Medial end is at the "tear drop". Inferior margin is at level of acetabular foramen. The centre of acetabular component is marked on the radiograph. This corresponds to the new centre of rotation of hip. Make an index mark above the previous mark at a distance equal to the amount of leg length correction required

Lateralized acetabulum on the other hand is seen with hypertrophic osteoarthritis particularly with medial osteophytes. This is identified if the tear drop is not immediately medial to the inferior border of the acetabulum. On the patient, in a surgical setting, the inferior border of the transverse acetabular ligament identifies the inferior border of the true acetabulum.

Superolateral migration is identified when placing the template leaves the supero-lateral portion of the cup uncovered by the bone. Medial reaming of the subchondral plate is helpful, in addition to using a low profile cup. The cup placement may be relatively vertical with an elevated rim liner in the superior position.

Femoral Templating

The sizing for the implant is done on the AP radiograph of hip with thigh. The radiograph should be taken with the femur in 15-20 degrees of internal rotation to have the correct profile of the bone including the neck length, offset and the resection level of the neck (Figs 6.5A to C).

In case of excessive and fixed deformity the templating may have to be done on the unaffected side, but this may not be accurate.

Choose the template size which:
- Matches the contour of proximal femur
- Fills it most completely proximally and fits distally
- Has space for cement all around for cemented stem fixation.

The center of rotation as determined by acetabular templating is marked on the X-ray plate. Using this as the reference point the femur is templated. The stem is centered along the neutral axis of the femur. Select appropriate neck length and offset which restores

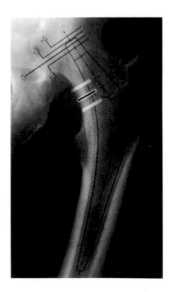

Fig. 6.5A: Femoral templating. Choose template size which matches contour of proximal femur. Fills it most completely. Keep space for cement in case of cemented implant. Select appropriate neck length which restores limb length and offset. Once neck length is selected, mark level of anticipated resection and measure distance from top of lesser trochanter-intraoperative guide. Template femur on lateral view to check for size. Measure canal diameter below the tip of femoral stem, to determine size of medullary plug, in case cemented stem

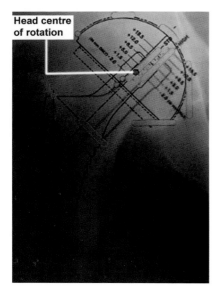

Head centre
of rotation

Fig. 6.5B: Femoral templating (Corail™ stem, J & J Depuy) The Corail stem is designed to seat in cancellous bone, and cortical contact should be avoided when templating. Select the appropriate template size that is smaller than the cortex in the proximal femur. The femoral template should be in line with the long axis of the femur and the neck resection line drawn at the point where the selected stem provides the desired amount of leg length. The vertical distance between the planned center of rotation of the acetabular component and the center of rotation of the femoral head constitutes the distance the leg length will be adjusted. The level of neck osteotomy depends on the stem size and the desired leg length, with the goal of using a non-skirted modular head to optimize range of motion prior to prosthetic impingement. To help properly position the template on the lateral radiograph, estimate the distance between the tip of the greater trochanter and the lateral shoulder of the prosthesis using the A/P radiograph (Figure C). Verify that the stem size chosen in the A/P plane also fits in the lateral plane. The lateral radiograph of a properly sized Corail implant will not exhibit cortical contact.

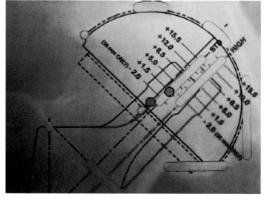

Fig. 6.5C: Offset requirement: The Corail Total Hip System implants are available with standard, high offset and varus options for all stem body sizes. Through templating and intraoperative trialing, determine which option restores proper offset by matching the cup's center of rotation with the desired head center of rotation

limb length and offset. Finally, mark the anticipated resection level and measure the distance from the top of lesser trochanter as the per-operative guide. Neck cuts are usually planned 1-2 cm above the lesser trochanter.

The center of femoral head is compared to the marked acetabular center of rotation. If the center of rotation of femur matches with that of the acetabulum then length and offset will be achieved without any modification. The neck resection level is marked through the template and the distance can be measured from the lesser trochanter. If the femoral center's vertical level is the same but more medial then increased femoral offset may be required, a few millimeters of which is only beneficial. If the femoral head center is vertically the same (as the acetabular center) but laterally placed means decreased femoral offset of the implant however is not desirable. This can be compensated by seating the component lower at the

CONSENT

Name of the patient: _____ Date: _____

Son / Wife / Daughter of: _____ Reg. No: _____

Address: _____ IP .No : _____

Operating Surgeon: _____ Tel. No. _____

1. I, _____, son / daughter / wife of

   _____, resident of

   _____, have been

   informed by the doctor that the clinical diagnosis of my disease is _____

   _____

2. I have been further informed by the doctor that the treatment planned for my disease is

   _____

3. I have been given the options to ask for any second opinion regarding the diagnosis or treatment.

4. I have been informed that after surgery, I will not be able to squat on the ground or sit cross-legged.

5. The risks of the surgery have been discussed with me in the language I understand. The major risks which have been discussed include:
   A. Infection
   B. Deep vein thrombosis and pulmonary embolism
   C. Anaesthetic risks

6. I have been given the opportunity to ask all questions and I have been satisfactorily answered.

7. I am aware that in the practice of medicine, other untoward / unexpected risks or complications not discussed may occur. I further understand that during the course of the proposed surgical procedure, unforeseen conditions may be revealed necessitating the performance of additional rectifying / modifying surgery.

8. The translation of the above has been made and explained to me in the language I best understand.

_____
Date of surgery

Signature of the patient / authorizing person
(with relation to the patient being mentioned)

Witnesses:

1. Name   Sign   Relationship

2. Name   Sign   Relationship

same time using a low neck cut and utilizing a longer head. This may require additional femoral reaming to have a 2 mm mantle for the cemented implant. There may be a problem in trying to achieve a perfect fill of femur in proximally coated implants which is essential. Alternatively a high offset implant design may be used. The recent modular designs have the option of changing the offset.

The modular implants with extra long neck lengths may have skirting which if present impinges in extremes of movement. Hence, the femoral neck resection level should be judiciously decided so that the usage of these implants with the extra long neck is avoided.

The planning of femoral entry point is also decided on the AP view of the hip. It is situated laterally by the side of or at the pyriformis fossa. The correct point is ascertained by extrapolating a line along the lateral wall of femur. The canal diameter and implant size is determined on the AP radiograph.

Templating would vary depending on the implant being planned viz. cemented, cementless proximally coated or cementless extensively coated implant. If cemented stem is being planned, a 2-3 mm gap is left for the cement mantle. With cementless 'extensively-coated implant' fixation is achieved distally. The stem should be in contact for several centimeters with the medial and lateral walls of the femoral canal.

In a patient with coxa vara use prosthesis with lower neck shaft angle or make a lower neck cut with and a long necked prosthesis. In patients with coxa valga use a high neck cut with a shorter neck length. A CDH implant may be used.

Consent for the Surgery (Total Hip Replacement)

Joint replacement is an irreversible procedure requiring certain changes in patient's life style. The consent taken should be a comprehensive one and should include this (particularly the inability to sit on the ground). Besides it should include the possibility of complications such as infection, deep vein thrombosis/pulmonary embolism and others because of existing co-morbidities in a patient. It is safer and sensible to be forthright in the beginning than trying to explain it subsequently. This is therefore called the 'informed consent' (Page no. 73). The document should be witnessed and counter signed preferably by a first degree relative.

Chapter Seven

Cemented Hip Replacement

Sir John Charnley first introduced cementing technique in Total Hip Arthroplasty (THA) for anchoring the implants in 1958 (Fig. 7.1). Bone cement currently used is a polymer of PMMA (polymethylmethacrylate) and MMA (methylmethacrylate). Its use is a part of a concept called the composite fixation (the metallic implant is stabilized in the bone by addition of cement).There is a mechanical interlock between the implant and the cement; the cement acting as a grout. It acts as elastic buffer and leads to optimal stress distribution to the bone.

The bone-cement polymer has many advantages:
- It gives immediate bio-mechanical stability to the construct
- Facilitates early weight bearing and rehabilitation
- It is cheap, easily available and in trained hands gives predictable result
- Antibiotics, combined with bone-cement are a local drug delivery system to reduce the risk of infection.

There are however few disadvantages in using the bone cement:
- It has an exothermic reaction when it cures and may devitalize adjacent bony tissue
- It is non-biodegradable
- It is weak in compression and torsion and hence may undergo fatigue fracture
- It is dissimilar from bone with no osteoinductive or osteoconductive property
- Breakdown particles generated induce chronic inflammatory and foreign body reaction leading to periprosthetic osteolysis and loosening of the implant, 'the particulate disease'.

Bone cement is available under various brand names. It is supplied as a 'two component system' a polymer powder in a plastic packing and a liquid in an ampoule (Fig. 7.2).

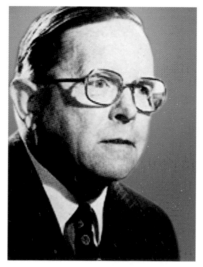

Fig. 7.1: Sir John Charnley

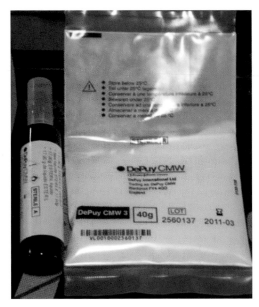

Fig. 7.2: Bone cement –liquid and powder

They are essentially of two types; high and low viscosity bone cements depending upon the duration of the liquid phase while curing.

Cementing Techniques

The cementing technique has evolved over the last five decades.

The *first generation* cement technique involved finger packing the cement when in a doughy state, no cement plug was used. The *second generation* cementing technique involved plugging the medullary canal, cleaning the cavity with pulsatile lavage and inserting cement in a retrograde fashion with cement gun. The *third generation* cementing technique involved vaccum mixing or centrifugation of the ingredients to reduce the size of the pores. The *fourth generation* technique besides all this included the use stem centralizer both proximally and distally.

An optimal cement fixation includes:
- A 2-3 mm cement-mantle, free of defects.
- A correctly centered femoral component in neutral alignment and optimum version.

CEMENTED HIP REPLACEMENT – ACETABULUM

Indications

- Arthritic hip over 60 years of age with adequate bone stock.
- Displaced fracture neck of femur in 60-70 years old.

Contra-indications (Relative)

- Poor acetabular bone stock
- Extensive bleeding of the acetabular surface
- Extensive cyst formation
- Weak cancellous bone following inflammatory pathology
- Protrusio hip
- Dysplastic hip
- Significant cardio-pulmonary disease.

Technique

Under hypotensive anesthesia usually epidural, the hip joint is exposed and dislocated, using any of the approaches (Figs 7.3A and B, 7.4A to E). We usually approach the joint using the anterolateral Sigma approach. Patient in lateral position the entire limb is cleaned and draped free in a stockinet up to the hip. An adhesive transparent film is applied at the site of the incision.

Once the hip joint is exposed the femoral head is dislocated and neck osteotomized. The femur is retracted away from the field (posteriorly in the anterolateral approach). The acetabular margin is identified and exposed using Hohmann's and pin retractors (Fig. 7.5). Overhanging capsular margin and labrum may be excised for better visibility. The transverse ligament is carefully preserved. The acetabulum is reamed with circumferential reamers

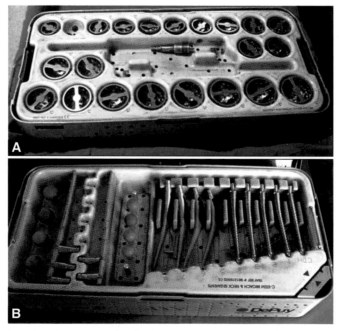

Figs 7.3A and B: *Instrumentation:* Instrument trays displaying (A) Acetabular reamers (B) Broaches, trial stems, trial heads and trial necks in that order from right

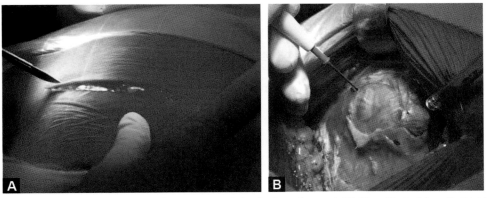

Figs 7.4A and B: *The anterolateral—Sigma approach (author's preference):* (A) The skin incision; Iliotibial band is cut in line with the superficial incision (Head of the patient is to the right), (B) A lazy-S incision on the anterolateral aspect of the trochanter is made and the cuff of tissue on the anterior aspect of the proximal femur is elevated. This includes the capsule, gluteus minimus and the anterior third of gluteus medius

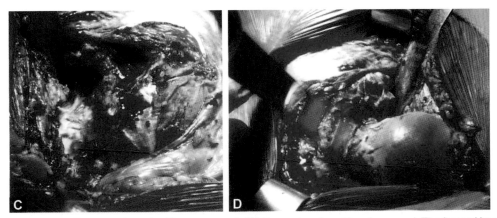

Figs 7.4C and D: *The anterolateral—Sigma approach:* (C) Femoral neck and head exposed. The femoral head in anterolateral approach is dislocated by flexing, adducting and externally rotating the lower limb, (D) The neck is then osteotomized. Osteotomy of the neck is about one finger breadth above the lesser trochanter. An osteotomy guide is useful in deciding the level

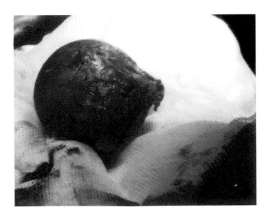

Fig. 7.4E: *The anterolateral—Sigma approach:* Osteotomized femoral head

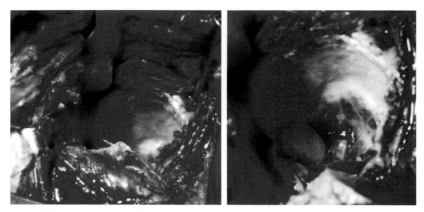

Fig. 7.5: *Acetabulum exposure and preparation*: Acetabulum is exposed using various retractors; the osteotomized femoral neck is retracted posteriorly

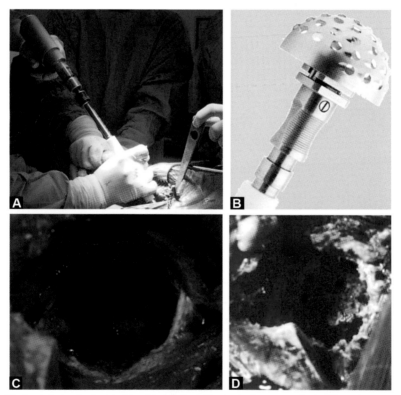

Figs. 7.6A to D: *Acetabular bed reaming*: Acetabulum is reamed progressively till oozing cancellous bone is exposed (A, B and C). The direction of reaming should be in line with the acetabulum. Multiple drill holes (D) Encourages better cement purchase on the bone

until the oozing cancellous bone is exposed. The medial cancellous bone is preserved. The reamers are numbered to accommodate the implant of the same size with 2-3 mm thick mantle of cement (Figs 7.6A to C).

Multiple drill holes are made into the dome of the acetabulum (Fig. 7.6D). The cavity is thoroughly lavaged, Water pick may be used to clear the debris. Trial cup is introduced on a cup holder and seated in correct orientation of 40° lateral opening and 15° anteversion (Fig. 7.7). High viscosity bone cement (e.g. CMW-1) is now prepared and once it becomes doughy is packed in the acetabulum. Excessive cement is removed from the inferior third. The cup is introduced on a cup holder and seated in correct orientation (Figs 7.8 and 7.9). The cement is pressurized by pushing in the cup in correct orientation using a pusher.

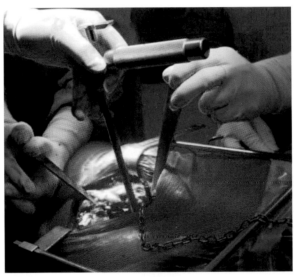

Fig. 7.7: *Trial acetabular implant placement*: Trial acetabular implant is seated using the orientation jig. The trial cup should fill the cavity completely

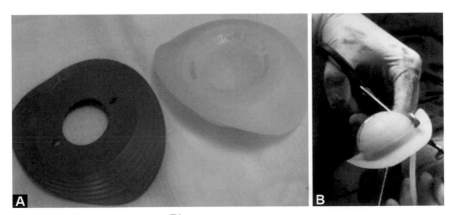

Fig. 7.8: *Definitive cup placement*: (A) Ogee™ cup (J & J, DePuy) and the blue template, the latter is used to map the surface of the acetabular opening, (B) Excessive flare of the cup is trimmed down so that the cup just fits into the acetabular cavity for effective pressurization of bone cement without 'bottoming out'

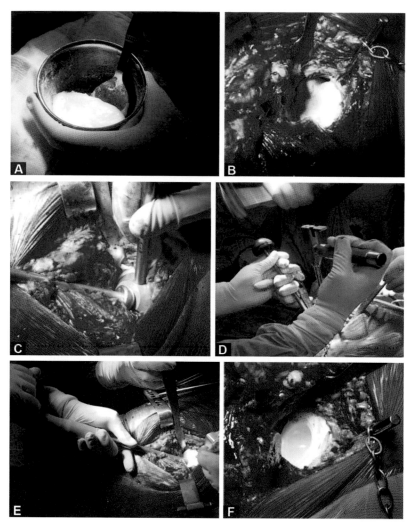

Figs. 7.9A to F: *Cementing the cup*: High viscosity bone cement may be mixed gently in a steel bowl (A). The dough is ready to use once it is does not stick to the glove any more. After cleaning and drying up the acetabulum a lump of cement dough is placed in the prepared acetabular bed (B). The cup on a holder is then introduced in optimal orientation (C). The pressurization is done by gently hammering the pusher and the holder (D). Excessive cement is curetted out and the position held with a pusher till the cement cures (E and F)

Extruded bone cement is removed particularly antero-inferiorly. Cups with peripheral flange (e.g. Ogee™ cup) allow even pressurization and prevent 'bottoming out' of the prosthesis in the acetabular cavity.

CEMENTED HIP REPLACEMENT – FEMUR

Once the hip joint is exposed and dislocated, using any of the approaches, the femoral neck is osteotomized at a slightly higher level than decided by templating. This holds true both for the arthritic hips as well as in fractures of the neck of femur. The acetabulum is then prepared. Femoral preparation is the next step. The proximal end of femur is levered out of the wound by gently rotating out the limb (externally for anterolateral approach) for good exposure.

Osteotomy of the Femoral Neck

Osteotomy of the neck is performed roughly at one to two finger breadths above the lesser trochanter or as pre-determined by templating using an oscillating saw (Fig. 7.10).

Canal Preparation

A point of entry is made just medial to the piriformis fossa (Fig. 7.11). The femur is held in external rotation, adduction and flexion in the anteriorly dislocated hip. This is how we normally dislocate the joint for hip replacement. When using the posterior approach for dislocating the hip the femur lies in internal rotation, adduction and flexion.

A box chisel may be used to pick up a chunk of good quality cancellous bone to open up the space. The same bone piece can be used as a bony plug before cementing the prosthesis. The femoral canal is then opened up with initial canal reamers (Fig. 7.12). The neck osteotomy may be finalized using a resection guide over the reamer (Fig. 7.13). A bony envelope is now created using a series of broaches progressively increasing in size. The broaches are designed to accommodate the said size implant and a 2 mm cement mantle all around it. The broaching should be in the neutral alignment and correct anteversion. The final broach should provide optimal metaphyseal fit and rotational stability. The broaching should save

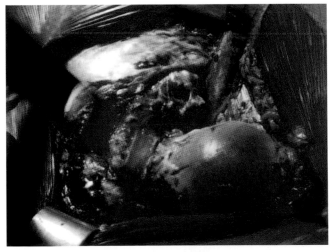

Fig. 7.10: *Femoral neck osteotomy:* Primary femoral neck osteotomy is performed at a level about a finger breadth above the lesser trochanter

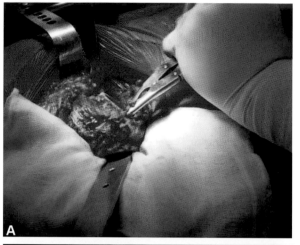

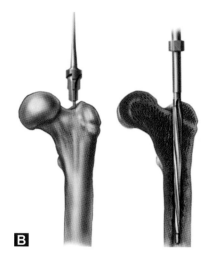

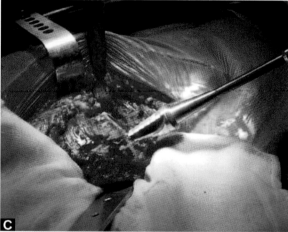

Figs 7.11A to C: *Femoral canal entry point*: Enter the femoral canal in line with the long axis of the femur in line with the pyriformis fossa. A nibbler or a starter drill may be used

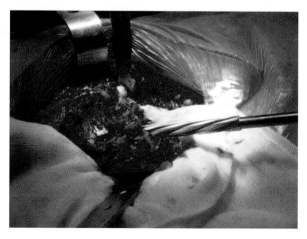

Fig. 7.12: *Canal reaming*: Incremental canal reaming is done to open up the isthmus. The final size is noted

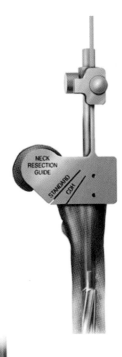

Fig. 7.13: Neck resection guide over the reamer may be used to assess true level of neck osteotomy

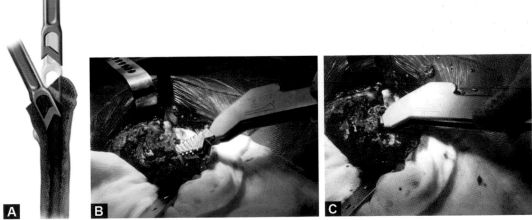

Figs 7.14A to C: *Canal broaching:* The entry point to the femoral canal is enlarged using the anterversion osteotome (box chisel) establishing 10 to 15 degrees of anteversion for proper implant alignment. Progressive broaching is done. To avoid varus malalignment or undersizing, the broaches are positioned laterally toward the greater trochanter

part of the cancellous bone for better inter-digitation of the cement into the bone and hence providing better shear strength (Fig. 7.14).

A trial reduction is then attempted using the final broach as a trial stem (Fig. 7.15).

A bone plug is now introduced 2-3 cm below the distal end of the planned implant. Alternatively it may be a plastic plug. This improves pressurization of cement into the bone and stops cement from migrating distally (Figs 7.16 and 7.17)

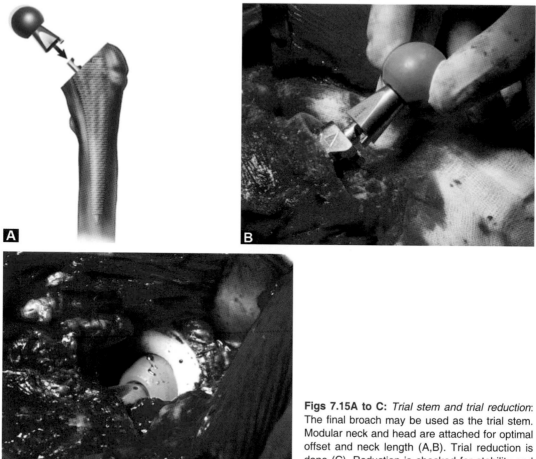

Figs 7.15A to C: *Trial stem and trial reduction*: The final broach may be used as the trial stem. Modular neck and head are attached for optimal offset and neck length (A,B). Trial reduction is done (C). Reduction is checked for stability and laxity

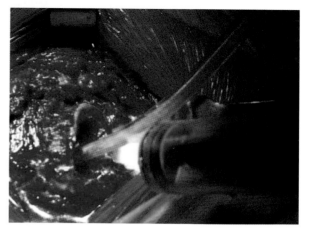

Fig. 7.16: *Femoral canal preparation*: The canal is thoroughly cleaned and lavaged

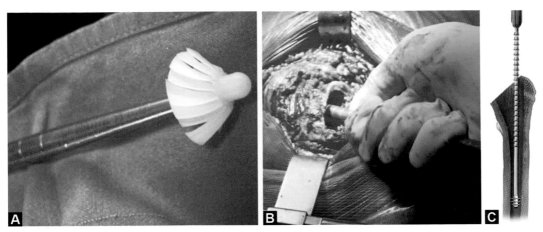

Figs 7.17A to C: *Bone plug:* A bone plug also called cement restrictor (Hardinge restrictor) is introduced at least 2-3 cm below the tip of the final implant (A,B,C). Measurement of the same is very important

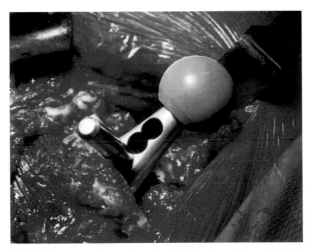

Fig. 7.18: *Trial stem with modular head:* Trial stem with modular head is introduced and joint reduced once more and stability checked

Trial stem is now fixed and a trial reduction redone. The level of stem insertion can be assessed (Fig. 7.18).

Free cancellous bone is then washed out and any loose tissue and debris removed using pulse lavage. This also reduces the incidence of fat embolism. The cavity is then packed with a gauge soaked with hydrogen peroxide.

Bone cement, preferably mixed by vacuum centrifugation is then introduced into the femoral canal with a cement gun. The cement used is a low–viscosity bone cement (e.g.

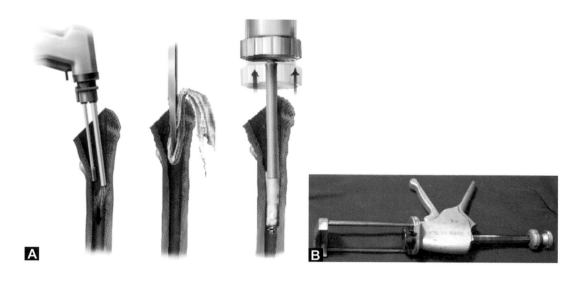

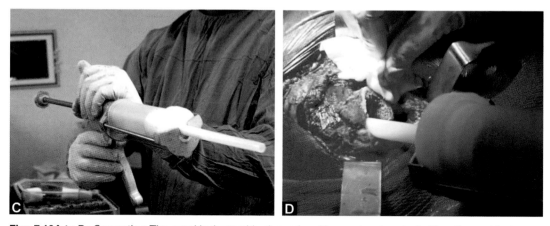

Figs 7.19A to D: *Cementing:* The canal is thoroughly cleaned and lavaged and packed with saline and hydrogen peroxide soaked roller gauge (A). Low viscosity bone cement is loaded in a cement gun and introduced in a retrograde fashion into the femoral canal after removing the pack (A,B,C,D)

CMW 3). The cavity is filled from the bottom to the top. High-viscosity cement (CMW 1) can alternatively be introduced using the manual technique. This is done over a suction cannula in the femoral cavity to suck out collective fluid and blood.

Once the cement becomes doughy, the femoral stem on a centralizer is introduced into the canal. The stem is inserted in its neutral alignment and appropriate version without

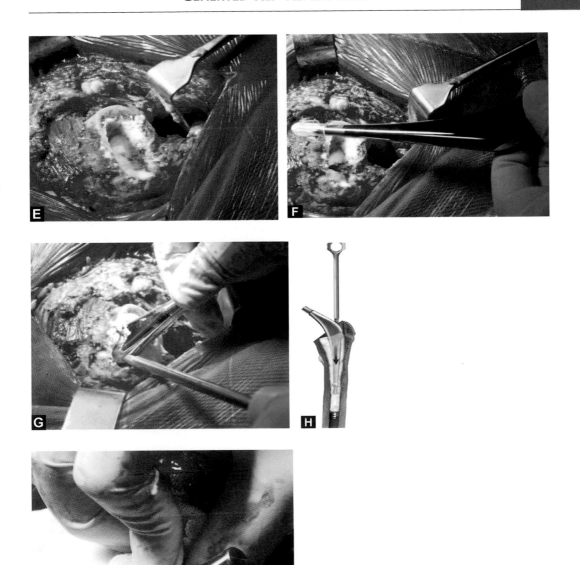

Figs 7.19E to I: *Cementing:* The definitive stem with centralizer is now introduced in correct version and alignment. No toggle is permitted as it will create voids in the cement mantle (E,F,G,H,I)

any toggle. Once the stem is inside the cement it should not be moved to correct the version or alignment as it creates voids in the cement mantle making it weak and prone to fracture (Fig 7.19).

The trial head is seated followed by trial reduction. Once a satisfactory size of neck length is decided the definitive head is sealed and joint reduced (Fig. 7.20).

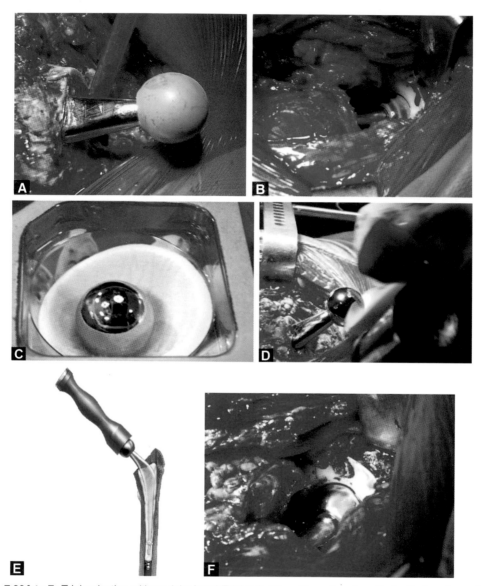

Figs 7.20A to F: *Trial reduction with modular head*: Trial reduction with modular head is finally done to confirm the size of the same (A,B). Definitive head of the selected size is snap fitted and joint reduced (C,D,E,F)

Radiographic Evaluation of Cement Mantle

Barrack et al. proposed a grading system (A to D) to assess the quality of cementing around the femoral stem. This should be done on the immediate post-operative radiograph (Figs 7.21 and 7.22).

A: Complete filling of the proximal diaphysis and difficulty in distinguishing cortex from the cement (white-out).

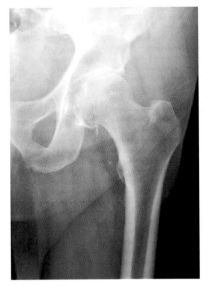 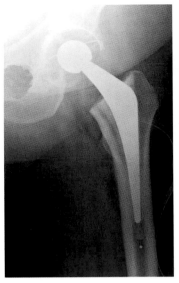

Fig. 7.21: Pre-op X-ray   **Fig. 7.22:** Post op X-ray - cemented THR

B: A near complete filling of the diaphysis; it being possible to distinguish between the cortex and the cement in some areas.

C1: An incomplete cement mantle in the proximal portion of the diaphysis, with greater than 50% of cement bone interface demonstrating radiolucencies.

C2: Mantle thickness less than 1mm or implant apposition against the cortex.

D: Gross deficiencies in the mantle, such as no cement distal to the implant tip or multiple large voids.

Type C and D are prone to early failure.

Chapter Eight

Cementless
Total Hip Replacement

Bone ingrowth with osseointegration of cementless implants in total hip replacement is now an established technique of implant fixation (Fig. 8.1). Cementless acetabular fixation is becoming popular because it is easy to implant and has reliable long term performance. The modular liner permits better stability. Fixation of the acetabular socket can be augmented with screws, if need be. The femoral stems also have a good performance; however there is some debate about certain features like the stem geometry; the type and the extent of porous coating, etc. (Fig. 8.2).

The cementless femoral stem may be extensively porous coated or proximally porous coated (Fig. 8.3). The immediate aim of surgery is to achieve axial and rotational stability by 4-5 cm of press-fit contact. The currenly available porous coated stems include a wide variety of designs; may be mono bloc or modular; the alloy used may be cobalt-chrome , titanium or composite; the surface treatment may be sintered beads, plasma spray, titanium fiber metal, corundumization or calcium–phosphate bioceramics. The cementless prosthesis is now being used in all bone types. However when used in Dorr type C femur one requires to use a thicker prosthesis because of the wide canal size which is a stiffer implant, all the

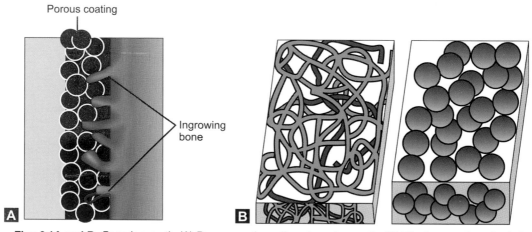

Figs 8.1A and B: *Bone in growth*: (A) Porous coating allows bone in growth. (B) Titanium mesh and cobalt chrome beads are two common ways to achieve the same

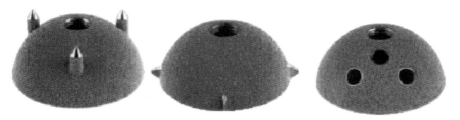

Fig. 8.2: *Cementless cups*: Various modes of primary fixation are available with modern cementless cups

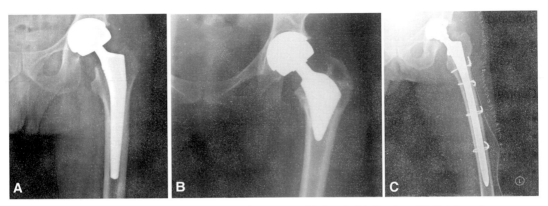

Figs. 8.3A to C: Radiographs of cementless stems (A) Corail (B) Proxima (C) Solution stem

more if it is made up of cobalt-chrome. This may lead to thigh pain and excessive proximal stress shielding. The proximally coated implants have a bulky proximal part with a narrow and flexible distal segment; this permits the loading of proximal femur and prevents proximal stress shielding.

Cementless Hip Replacement-Acetabulum

Predictable fixation of cementless cup involves the implant and the host biologic response. The implant should have a biologically friendly surface, intimate host-bone- implant apposition and rigid stability. Special instrumentation is required for the same (Fig. 8.4).

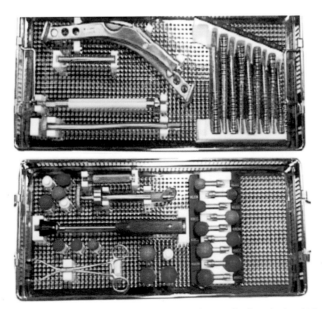

Fig. 8.4: *Instrumentation:* An array of instruments is required and should be available besides the general trauma set

Indications

- Primary arthroplasty in patients preferably with healthy local bony tissue and adequate pelvic support.

Contra-indications

- Severe metabolic bone disease, e.g. Osteomalacia, severe osteoporosis
- Irradiated bone
- Local metastasis
- Paget's disease.

Surgical Steps

The acetabulum is exposed circumferentially using any of the approaches. We prefer the antero-lateral approach as it permits good visualization of the acetabulum without endangering vital neurovascular structures. It is easier to place the cup in correct ante-version and inclination through this approach (Figs 8.5 to 8.8).

With the acetabulum once exposed the labrum is completely excised and peri-acetabular osteophytes removed (Fig. 8.9). The pulvinar is removed and the medial aspect of the acetabulum identified. Any osteophyte if present here is nibbled or reamed directly medially till all of it is removed and true medial wall identified. There after the acetabular reaming is carried out in correct anteversion and inclination (40° of abduction and 10°-20° of anteversion). The reaming is continued with sequential circumferential reamers till bleeding cancellous bone is exposed without breaching the medial integrity (Fig. 8.10). The acetabular bed is inspected for sub-chondral cysts and defects which are to be bone grafted. The acetabulum is usually under-reamed by 1 or 2 mm for press fit.

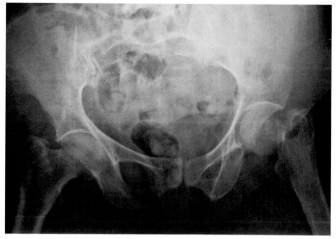

Fig. 8.5: *Preoperative radiograph*: Preoperative radiograph showing fracture neck of femur with ipsilateral reduced joint space. The patient was planned for cementless THR

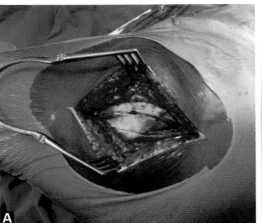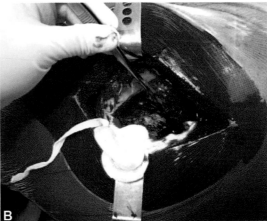

Figs. 8.6A and B: (A) *Skin incision using the anterolateral-Sigma approach (author's preference)*: (A) The Iliotibial band is cut in line with the incision, (B) Elevating the cuff of tissue on the anterior aspect of the proximal femur. This includes the capsule, gluteus minimus and the anterior third of gluteus medius

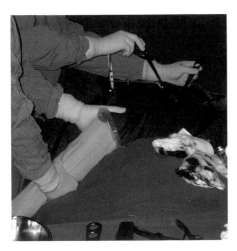

Fig. 8.6C: The femoral head in anterolateral approach is dislocated by flexing adducting and externally rotating the lower limb

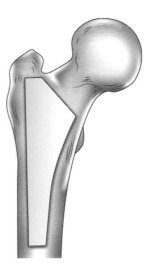

Fig. 8.7A: *Osteotomy femoral neck*: The neck is then osteotomized. Here since the patient has fracture of the neck of femur the osteotomy was performed before delivering out the head. Osteotomy of the neck is about one finger breadth above the lesser trochanter. The neck osteotomy guide is useful in deciding the level

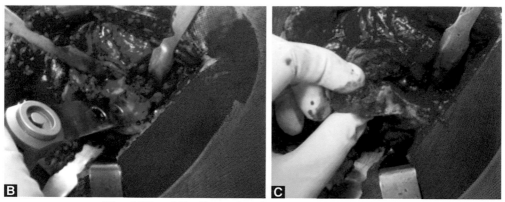

Figs 8.7B and C: Femoral neck osteotomized and sliver of bone removed (in fracture neck of femur)

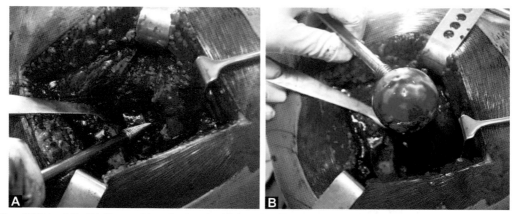

Figs 8.8A and B: (A) *Femoral head extraction/dislocation*: Femoral head being removed using myomectomy screw, (B) Femoral head dislocated out

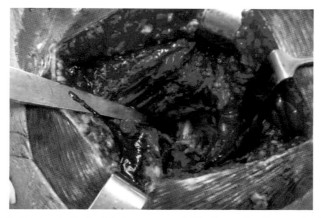

Fig. 8.9: *Acetabular exposure*: Acetabulum exposed. The femur has been retracted posteriorly

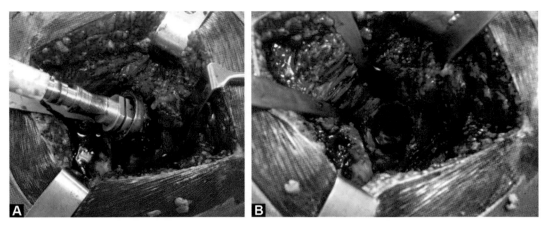

Figs 8.10A and B: (A) *Acetabular reaming*: Incremental acetabular reaming is done to accommodate the implant of appropriate size. The last reamer is undersized by 1-2 mm compared to the implant for press-fit, (B) Prepared acetabular bed

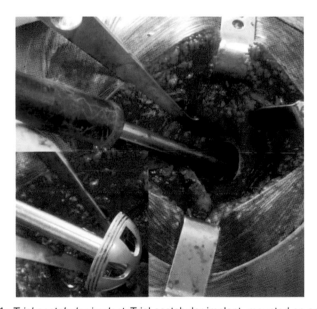

Fig. 8.11: *Trial acetabular implant*: Trial acetabular implant mounted on an inserter

Trial prosthesis is then inserted and stability checked (Fig. 8.11). Acetabular size once selected, the definitive implant is seated in correct inclination and version. Socket holders are useful in getting the placement right (Figs 8.12A and B). The fixation may be augmented with screws in the safe zone in case the socket is felt to be less than perfectly secure (Fig. 8.12C).

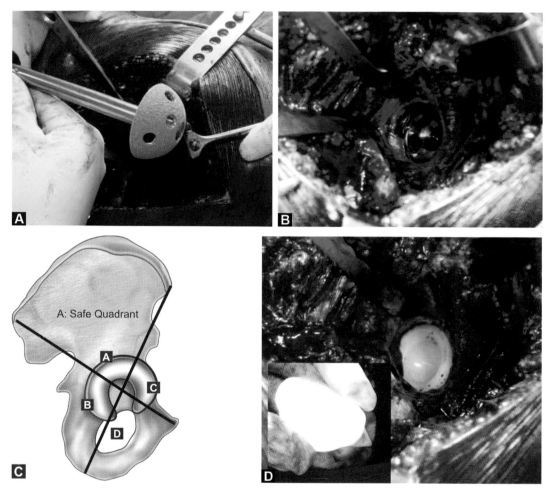

Figs 8.12A to D: *Definitive acetabular shell*: (A) Definitive shell mounted on a inserter, (B) Definitive acetabular shell seated (C). If the fixation is less than satisfactory additional reinforcement is achieved using screws in the safe quadrant, (D) Definitive acetabular cup (liner) seated

The liner is now inserted which may be a trial component initially and is then replaced with the final implant after femoral preparation (Fig. 8.12D). The liner used may have a design that incorporates an elevation over a portion of the circumference of the rim which may be rotated superiorly or posteriorly for better joint stability to offset any incorrection in the placement of shell. Other design options completely re-orient the opening face of the socket by up to 20 degrees and still other lateralizes the hip center.

Cementless Hip Replacement-Femur

Indications

- Primary arthroplasty in patients preferably with Dorr type A and B femur
- Previous surgery with bone defect (s)/implant removal.

Contra-indications

- Severe osteoporosis
- Where initial fixation is a concern
- Where proximal femoral osteotomy is required proximally coated stems are contraindicated
- Deformed proximal femur.

Surgical Steps

The hip joint is exposed using either of the approaches. The author's choice is the anterolateral approach. Once the acetabular reaming and prosthetic implantation is complete femoral preparation is started. The surgical steps are:

- Reaming
- Broaching and trial implant fixation with trial reduction.
- Definitive implant fixation and joint reduction.

Reaming

The proximal femur is exposed by levering it out on a trochanteric lever and rotating externally for anteriorly dislocated hip. Incremental reaming in a serial fashion is done to achieve the appropriate fit at the isthmus for initial stability for extensively coated stems (Figs 8.13 and 8.14). This is particularly required for prosthetic design with straight stem. The pilot hole is made within the trochanteric fossa at the insertion of piriformis tendon using a starting reamer or a high speed burr. The first reamer should pass easily and stay centered in the hole, if it does not the hole should be reoriented. Medial and anterior entry points should be avoided. The author prefers version-osteotome (box-chisel) as the first step to remove bone from proximal metaphysis in the desired version for the final femoral implant. Subsequent reaming is done with hand held reamers progressively increasing in size to within 2 mm of the templated size. Power reaming may be required if the isthmus is very narrow. The aim is to achieve adequate press fit for initial stabilization.

The final reamer size should be checked with the trial implant for the actual distal dimension. In Corail^{TM} system, used here, reaming is not a part of the standard surgical technique as it is based on the principle of bone impaction.

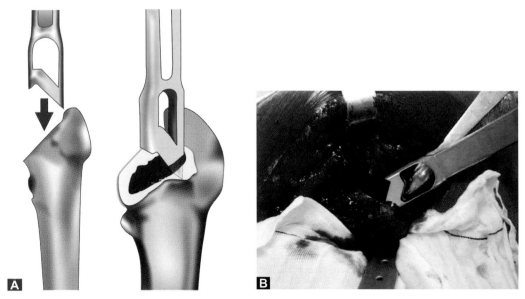

Figs 8.13A and B: *Femoral pilot hole*: In Corail™ uncemented hip system the version osteotome is used to make a pilot hole at the pyriformis fossa followed by the broaches

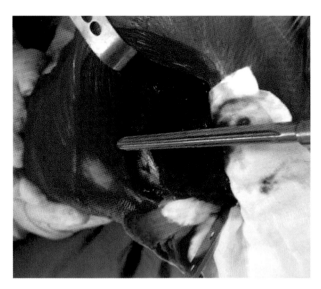

Fig. 8.14: *Femoral canal reaming*: Initial femoral reaming of femoral isthmus is required in most of the hip systems however the Corail™ (J and J-De Puy), described here, is based on the principle of compressing and compacting the cancellous bone and hence this step is not recommended

Broaching

Metaphyseal broaching is performed to accommodate the implant's proximal geometry (Fig. 8.15). The broaching is begun with smallest sized broach and increased progressively. It is to be matched to the size of the last reamer distally in extensively coated femoral stems. Broaching should be done in the correct anteversion as it cannot be corrected subsequently which will decide the final version while seating the implant.

If despite proper seating of the broach, there is excessive cancellous bone medially further broaching to a higher size is done. On the other hand, if even the smallest broach cannot be completely seated the proximal medial endosteum is sculpted with a high-speed burr till full seating can be arranged. The broach should be backed out repeatedly before final seating as it helps in better seating by removing the debris. Once the final seating of the broach is satisfactory a trial reduction is done with the appropriate size neck length (Fig. 8.16). The trial reduction should permit the use of at least one size shorter neck. So that if the definitive stem seating is tighter or prouder with the definitive prosthesis then the neck can be undersized.

The offset of the construct if need be can be increased by deep seating the final broach (may be by undersizing it) and then using a longer neck. The offset can be decreased by keeping the stem a little proud and using a short neck. However do not compromise on proximal fill and distal fit.

Stem Placement

The distal portion of the stem is seated in the medullary canal in appropriate anteversion. This may be done with impaction handles or manually. The stem is impacted with firm blows of the mallet. The stem should be observed to advance about 2 mm with each blow which gradually slows down. Full implant seating should be achieved. The sound at final seating is a sharper high pitched tone compared to a hollow note in the beginning (Fig. 8.17).

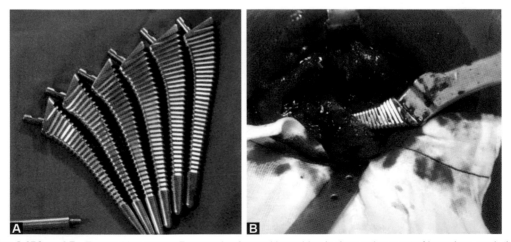

Figs 8.15A and B: *Femoral broaching:* Progressive femoral broaching is done using a set of broaches, such that the distal stem and proximal femur accommodate a well fitting implant. A change in the sound quality produced by hammering is noticed as the appropriate size is reached. The entire broach should be well seated (A) broaches of various sizes, (B) broaching in progress

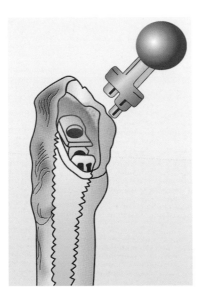

Fig. 8.16: *Trial femoral implant*: In the Corail™ system used here the correct size broach is used as a trial stem. The modular head and neck is chosen for correct offset and length

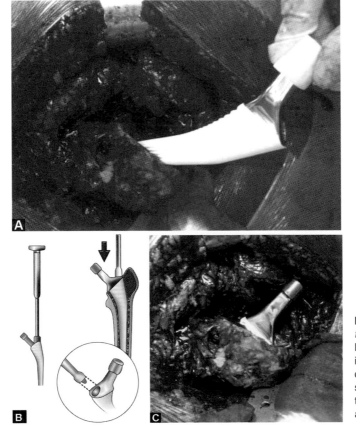

Figs 8.17A to C: *Definitive femoral implant seated*: Definitive cementless stem is introduced into the femoral canal in correct version gently sliding it into the femoral canal till appropriate insertion is achieved

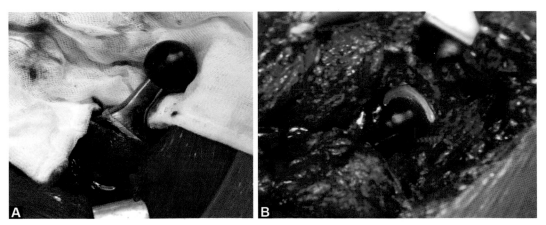

Figs 8.18A and B: *Trial head and reduction*: Trial femoral head is reinserted and reduction is tried again for stability in all directions and tissue laxity. Suitable adjustments are made if need be

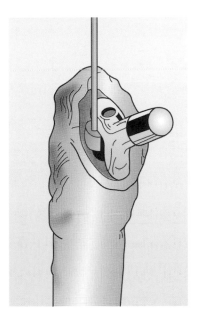

Fig. 8.19: *Proximal femoral grafting*: Graft is packed around the definitive stem to obliterate the dead space

If for some reason the seating is higher than that of the expected final seating a small size neck may be used. If this is not available or not useful then the implant is removed. The implant and reamer sizes are physically checked and reaming and broaching repeated. Care is taken not to over-ream as the distal stability would be jeopardized.

Once the stem placement is satisfactory an appropriate size trial head–neck is seated, reduction achieved and checked for stability (Fig. 8.18). Any gap around the proximal prosthesis and the bone is filled with bone graft (Fig. 8.19). The trial head is removed and is

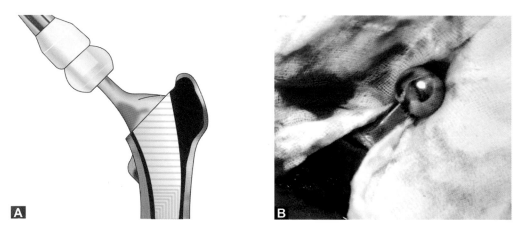

Figs 8.20A and B: *Definitive femoral head*: Definitive femoral head is then snap fitted over the stem

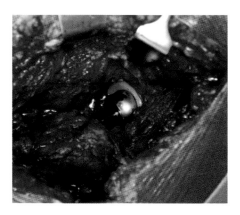

Fig. 8.21: Hip joint reduced, just before wound closure

Fig. 8.22: Pre-op and Post op X-ray THR cementless

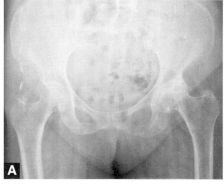
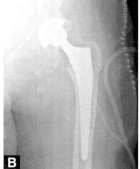

replaced by definitive implant of the same size and appropriate taper fit (Figs 8.20 to 8.22). The joint is reduced and checked for stability. The wound is closed in layers over a negative suction drain and aseptic dressing done.

Chapter Nine

Hemiarthroplasty Hip

Hemiarthroplasty for the hip is a commonly done procedure for fracture of neck of femur in the elderly population.

Indications

1. **Femoral neck fracture** (preferred over osteosynthesis) in patients with:
    - Physiologic age more than 70 yrs.
    - Poor general health that would make second surgery dangerous.
    - Pathologic fracture with healthy uninvolved acetabulum in elderly patient.
    - Parkinson's disease, hemiplegia, or other neurological disease.
    - Severe osteoporosis (as diagnosed with loss of primary trabeculae in femoral head using Singh's index).
    - Less than optimal closed reduction of fracture neck of femur.
    - Displaced fracture which is several days old.
2. Pre-existing hip disease (e.g. avascular necrosis of femoral head) not involving the acetabulum.

    It is preferred over total hip replacement in cases of:
1. Abductor muscle weakness or deficiency.
2. As a salvage procedure in massive acetabular deficiencies particularly in revision total hip replacements.

Contraindications

These include:
- History of pre-existing sepsis (absolute contraindication for any joint replacement).
- Bipolar hip replacement in young patients—in view of excessive wear rate of the plastic liner.
- Pre-existing disease of the acetabulum.
- Dysplastic hip with a high sourcil slope (sourcil is a radiodense subchondral bone of the weight-bearing dome of the acetabulum).

Types of Hemiarthroplasty

According to the prosthetic head type used:
  i. Unipolar, e.g. Austin Moore/Thompson Prosthesis (Fig. 9.1)
  ii. Bipolar (Fig. 9.9)

According to the femoral stem fixation:
  i. Cemented
  ii. Cementless.

Prosthetic femoral head size should match the natural femoral head size; if it is too large equatorial contact may be tight and may not permit reduction of the joint or else may cause painful restriction of the movements. If the head is too small polar contact occurs leading to early erosive and degenerative changes in the acetabulum due to stress concentration eventually requiring an early change of the acetabular surface.

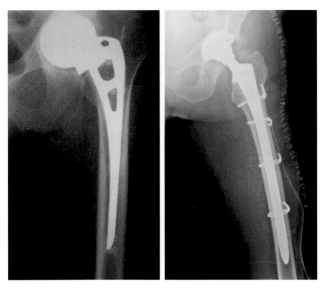

Fig. 9.1: Radiograph of Austin Moore prosthesis *in situ* showing erosion of acetabular cartilage. Treated by revision total hip arthroplasty

The neck length should be optimal; if excessively long it may lead to difficulty in reduction, limb lengthening and excessive pressure on the acetabulum leading to early wear of acetabular cartilage.

The neck length should be such that the distance between the greater trochanter and the center acetabulum and the distance between the lesser trochanter and the center of acetabulum is restored. This recreates the natural limb length and abductor lever arm.

Cemented femoral stem like in cemented total hip replacement is preferred in patients with 'stove pipe' (Dorr type C) femur. Dorr type A femurs are good candidates for cementless stem fixation. However, patients with poor cardiac risk who cannot tolerate cementing induced hypotension and also those with poor surgical risk are considered for cementless fixation. A good ambulator with stovepipe femur may have thigh pain with cementless stem because of excessive stiffness of a thick implant.

Gilbert and Bateman (1974) were the first to use bipolar prosthesis. The rationale for such use was to minimize damage to the acetabular cartilage by distributing the shear forces at two levels, the inner and outer bearings. Bipolar designs provide greater overall range of motion compared to unipolar designs. However, the degree of inner bearing motion decreases with time. The current designs provide eccentric placement of metallic and polyethylene cups to avoid fixation in varus and fracture of polyethylene part or dislocation. Due to the risk of polyethylene debris induced osteolysis many surgeons prefer unipolar prosthesis especially in young patients.

Complications that may be encountered are:
- Erosion of articular cartilage (Fig. 9.1)
- Acetabular migration especially in soft bones like rheumatoid arthritis.
- More osteolysis due to higher polyethylene wear debris compared to total hip replacements, hence bipolar arthroplasty is to be avoided in young patients.

Surgical Steps

Under anesthesia, patient usually in lateral position, the entire limb is cleaned and draped free in a stockinet up to the hip. An adhesive transparent film is applied at the level of the incision. The hip joint and fracture is exposed, using any of the approaches. We usually approach the joint using the anterolateral approach (Fig. 9.2). The fractured femoral neck is osteotomized roughly at one finger breadth above the lesser trochanter or as per the level decided upon at templating. The femoral head and acetabulum are then easily exposed once the femur is retracted away from the field (posteriorly in the anterolateral approach) (Fig. 9.3). The head is delivered out using a myomectomy screw or if need be is removed piece-meal (Figs 9.4 and 9.5). The femoral head size is measured using the head gauge. The largest size of the gauge through which the head cannot pass is the correct size (Fig. 9.6).

Canal Preparation

The proximal femur is exposed and elevated using a trochanteric lever. The femoral shaft is held in adduction, flexion and external rotation in anteriorly dislocated hip. A point of entry is made just medial to the piriformis fossa. In a posteriorly dislocated hip the femur

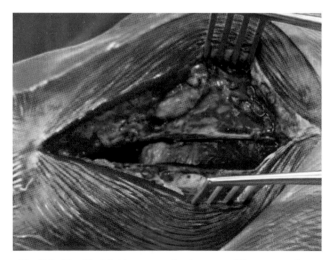

Fig. 9.2: The hip joint is exposed using any of the approaches.
Here the joint is exposed using the anterolateral approach

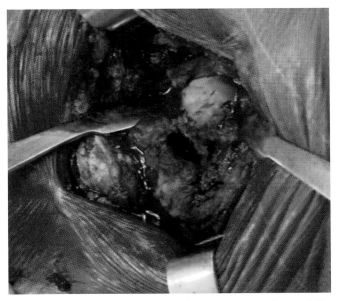

Fig. 9.3: The proximal femur and the fracture is exposed through the anterolateral approach. The fracture neck of femur is visible

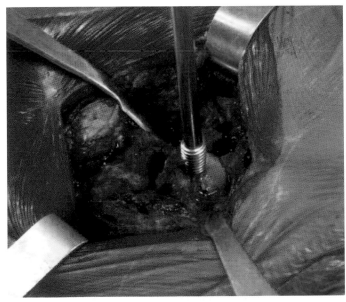

Fig. 9.4: The femoral head being extracted using a myomectomy screw

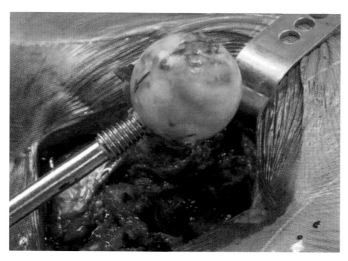

Fig. 9.5: Femoral head dislocated out

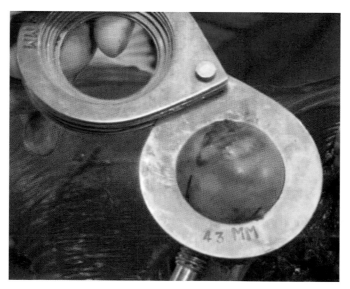

Fig. 9.6: Sizing the femoral head. Here the size accepted is 43 mm

lies in internal rotation, adduction and flexion. A box chisel may be used to pick-up a chunk of good quality cancellous bone to open up the space. The same bone piece can be used as a bony plug in femoral diaphysis before cementing the prosthesis. The femoral canal is then opened up with initial canal reamers (Fig. 9.7). A bony envelope is now defined using a series of broaches progressively increasing in size (Fig. 9.8). In cemented hip the broaches

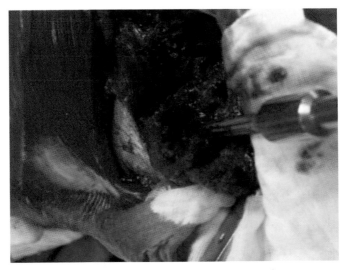

Fig. 9.7: The femoral canal being reamed

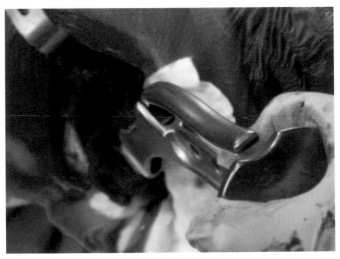

Fig. 9.8: Broaching the proximal femur

are designed to accommodate the said size implant and a 2 mm cement mantle all around it. In cementless stem the implant is pressfit. The reaming should be in the neutral alignment and desired anteversion. The final broach should provide optimal metaphyseal fit and rotational stability. The broaching should save part of the cancellous bone for better interdigitation of the cement onto the bone and hence better shear strength. A trial reduction may now be carried out.

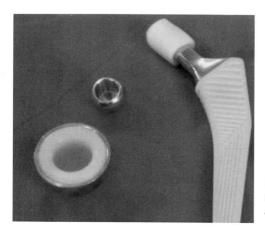

Fig. 9.9: The components of a bipolar hip: The bipolar head with the plastic liner, the modular femoral head and the femoral stem (Corail™).

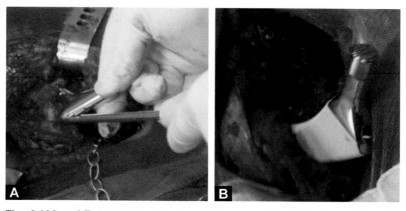

Figs 9.10A and B: Introducing the femoral stem cemented (A) and cementless (B)

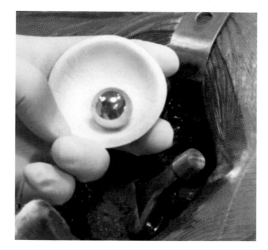

Fig. 9.11: The definitive head. Definitive femoral stem already seated

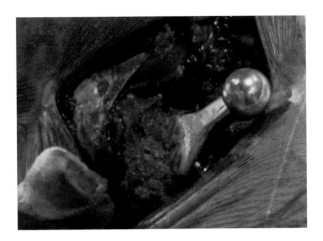

Fig. 9.12: The definitive modular head. Seated on the femoral stem

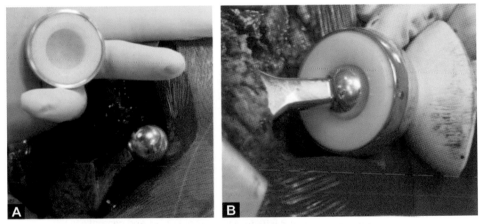

Figs. 9.13A and B: The bipolar head being mounted

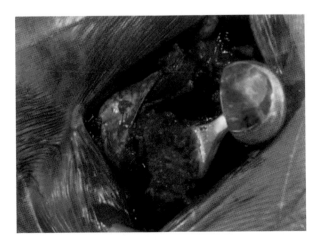

Fig. 9.14 : The final construct

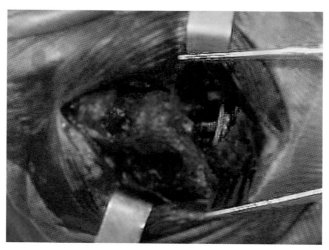

Fig. 9.15: Joint reduced and ready for closure

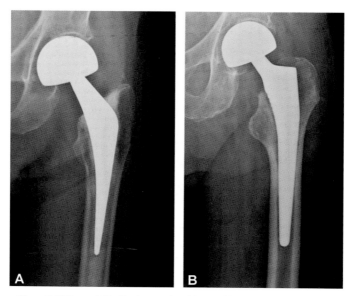

Figs. 9.16A and B: Postoperative X-rays bipolar hip arthroplasty cemented (C-stem^TM) and cementless (Corail^TM)

A bone plug is now introduced 2-3 cm below the distal end of the implant planned in case of a cemented stem. Alternatively, in cemented stem placement a bony or a plastic plug may be used. Free cancellous bone is now washed out and any loose tissue and debris removed using pulse lavage. This also reduces the incidence of fat embolism. The cavity is then packed with a gauge soaked with hydrogen peroxide. Bone cement is then introduced inside with a cement gun. The cement used is low-viscosity bone cement (e.g. CMW-3) the cavity is filled from the bottom to the top. High-viscosity cement (CMW-1) dough can alternatively be introduced using the manual technique for packing. This is done over an infant feeding tube to suck out collected fluid from the bottom of the cavity. Once the cement becomes stiffer, the femoral stem on a centralizer is introduced into the canal using a pusher. The stem is inserted in its neutral alignment and appropriate version without any toggle. Once the stem is inside the cement it should not be moved as it is known to create voids in the cement mantle making it prone to early failure.

A cementless stem of appropriate size when used is seated in correct version and depth (Fig. 9.10).

Trial femoral head is now seated and trial reduction achieved. Appropriate length of femoral neck is chosen for stability and length. Trial head is replaced by definitive head (Figs 9.11 and 9.12). The bipolar metal head of the correct size (as chosen by measurement with the head gauge) with a plastic liner is now mounted on the prosthetic head (Figs 9.13 and 9.14). The joint is then reduced and checked for stability (Fig. 9.15). The wound is closed in layers over a negative suction drain.

The femoral stem fixation may be cemented or cementless (Fig. 9.16).

Chapter Ten

Postoperative Management and Rehabilitation

Immediate Postoperative Care

The patient after the surgery is shifted to the recovery/high dependency unit (HDU) for postoperative monitoring (Fig. 10.1). The patient is transported in supine position with the operated limb abducted by a pillow. Strapping should be avoided as it may lead to pressure sores at the ankle. The patient is permitted some degrees of flexion at the hip provided the preoperative stability was good. He/she may also be permitted to lie in the lateral position on the nonoperative side while maintaining the pillow between the knees. Early turning in bed prevents bed-sore formation and most of the patients are more comfortable this way. The patient is encouraged ankle and toe mobilization in bed as soon as motor function recovers. An air-mattress may be used to prevent bed sores (Fig. 10.1).

In the recovery/HDU the patient is connected to the monitor using ECG leads, SpO_2 probe, BP cuff, etc. A continuous monitoring of pulse, SpO_2, BP, respiration and cardiac activity is done. The patient is also monitored for urine output, soakage and drain output.

Continuous analgesics are started for pain management. This may be done using an epidural infusion (Fig. 10.2) of analgesic solution (local anesthetics with/without fentanyl, tramadol, etc.) or through intravenous analgesics as infusion or as patient controlled analgesia (PCA). The dosage of infusion is adjusted according to the pain response which is evaluated regularly using the visual analog score (VAS) card (on a scale of 1 to 10) (Fig. 10.3). The patient is also regularly assessed for blood pressure and weakness or numbness

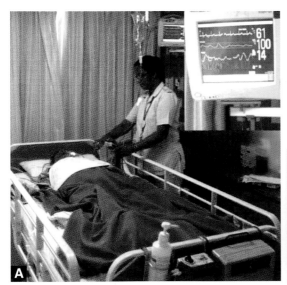
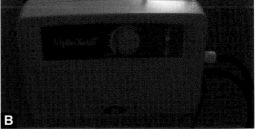

Figs 10.1A and B: Patient in ICU bed connected monitoring devices: (A) Patient being monitored, (B) Air mattress control

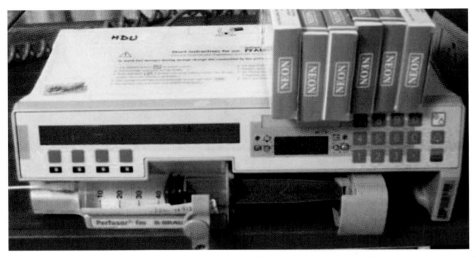

Fig. 10.2: Post-operative analgesia- infusion pump: (a) Epidural sensoricaine/ clonidine infusion (connected to epidural catheter), (b) iv fentanyl infusion (connected to intravenous cannula)

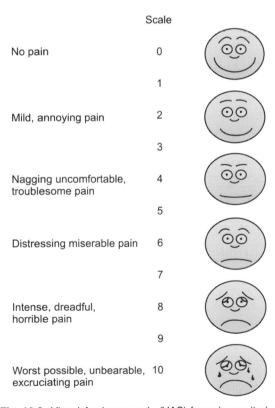

	Scale	
No pain	0	
	1	
Mild, annoying pain	2	
	3	
Nagging uncomfortable, troublesome pain	4	
	5	
Distressing miserable pain	6	
	7	
Intense, dreadful, horrible pain	8	
	9	
Worst possible, unbearable, excruciating pain	10	

Fig. 10.3: Visual Analogue scale (VAS) for pain monitoring

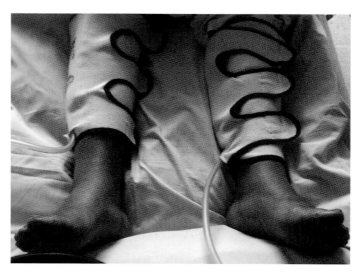

Fig. 10.4: DVT pump

of the lower limbs which may be because of overdose of anesthetics. The latter may very rarely be because of **epidural hematoma** particularly in patients with narrow spinal canal (due to degenerative spine) particularly those on blood thinners. This is a surgical emergency and needs to be decompressed immediately.

PCA is an infusion pump with narcotic analgesics controlled by a switch by the patient himself or herself. This has to be strictly followed. An over-zealous attendant may make the patient drowsy and stuprose, which can be dangerous and may even prove fatal. These pain control modalities are usually continued for 48 to 72 hours when the patient is put on suitable injectable/oral analgesics. The combination we prefer is NSAIDS, tramadol and paracetamol.

Intravenous antibiotics are started to cover both Gram negative and positive organisms. These are usually continued for 48 hours when it may be changed to oral antibiotics (we usually prefer the combination of Cefuroxime and Tobramicin). The patient may usually require parenteral antacids (proton pump inhibitors) and pro-kinetic agents in the immediate postoperative period. Thrombo-prophylaxis involves subcutaneous low molecular weight heparin (LMWH) which is started 12 hours after the surgery to avoid excessive bleeding both at the operative and the epidural site. The commonly used LMWH are enoxaparin and dalteparin. Deep veinthrombosis can be avoided using calf pump (Fig. 10.4).

Blood transfusion is decided depending upon the drainage and soakage. An average blood loss of about 150 ml is anticipated in the first 24 hrs following hip replacement in an average built patient. Transfusion of about two units of blood will be required if it is more. Use of packed RBCs minimizes transfusion reactions. Hb% and PCV values are checked the subsequent morning and additional transfusion is given if the hemoglobin is less than 10 gm%.

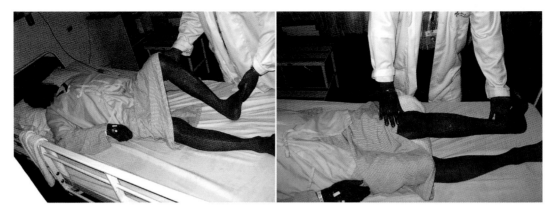

Fig. 10.5: In bed physiotherapy

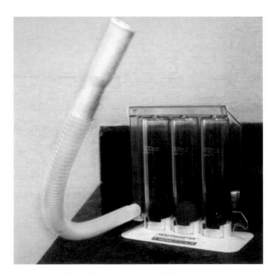

Fig. 10.6: Incentive Spirometery

The other blood tests routinely carried out on the first postoperative day are for serum electrolytes, blood urea and creatinine. The patient SpO_2 monitoring is important.

The suction drain is removed on the first post-operative day if the drainage is reasonable (less than 300 ml). In case the collection is more it may be retained for another 24 hours. Strict aseptic precautions are adhered to while removing the drain and change of dressing.

The patient is started on physiotherapy in bed on the first postoperative same day. Static glutei, abductors and quadriceps exercises are started. The patient is encouraged to prop up and chest physiotherapy is initiated (Incentive spirometry) (Fig. 10.6). Besides this he/she is taught to perform ankle pumps.

If all the parameters are within the normal range the patient is shifted to the ward on first postoperative day.

Management and Physiotherapy in the Ward

The diet is made regular as soon as the patient is ready. The bowel habits are regularized with laxatives/enema, if need be.The patient is put on oral antibiotics after 48-72 hours of injectables. The pain management continues in the ward. Parenteral analgesics are gradually replaced by oral formulations. Besides NSAIDs we prefer tramadol/paracetamol combination. The associated nausea and gastritis is managed accordingly.

The wound is inspected and the dressing changed in case of significant spotting/soakage.

In the ward physiotherapy is continued and the patient gradually starts to get to the daily routine of activities.

In bed supervised physiotherapy is done twice a day (Fig. 10.6). The exercises are continued and hip and knee flexion (slides) gradually increased. The patient is made to sit up in the bed and also with the legs hanging by the side of the bed. The patient is advised to strictly continue the abduction pillow and to not lie on the operated side for preferably six weeks and a minimum of three weeks.

On the second or the third postoperative day, depending on the comfort level, the patient is made to stand up and walk with walker (Fig. 10.7). Following cemented hip arthroplasty the patient is allowed complete weight bearing on the operated side. However following cementlesss or hybrid fixation partial weight-bearing is permitted. In thin built patients with very secure initial fixation of the component early complete weight bearing may be permitted.

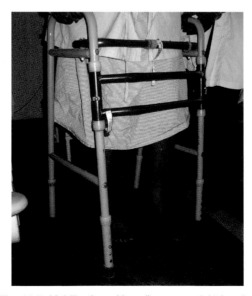

Fig. 10.7: Mobilisation with walker non weight bearing

The patient is permitted to visit the toilet by post-operative day three or four. A high western commode seat is used. This has to continue for three months.

The patient is discharged from the hospital on post-op day five. In case of bilateral hip replacement the patient goes home on postoperative day eight.

Care at Home and Follow-up

The oral antibiotics are continued up till postoperative day 5-7 depending on existing co-morbidities. The analgesics and other supportive medications are weaned off depending on patient's requirement. Patient continues supervised physiotherapy at home as before. The walker continues for a total of 3 to 4 weeks following cemented hip replacement when the patient graduates to a stick in the contralateral hand to the operated hip. Stair climbing is encouraged at around 4 weeks. All this is delayed in cementless hip replacement till solid fixation of the implant occurs which is about 6-12 weeks.

The patient follows-up at two weeks from surgery for suture removal and then again at six weeks for re-evaluation and radiological assessment (for cementless/hybrid hips). At that time a graduated increase in weight bearing is permitted to patients with cementless/hybrid hips.

By the end of three months the patient is usually off all forms of support.

Chapter Eleven

Complications following THR

The average mortality in total hip arthroplasty is about 1.2%. Postoperative complications are more common in older patients. Therefore careful evaluation and clinical judgment must be used to determine the physiological age of the patients. Poor outcomes and complications are related more to co-morbidities. Some complications of total hip replacement are inherent to any major orthopedic surgery, these include:
- Hemarthrosis/Hematoma
- Infection
- Neurovascular injuries
- Urinary tract infection
- Deep Vein Thrombosis/Pulmonary embolism.

Other complications of total hip replacement are specifically related to the procedure, these are:
- Limb length discrepancy
- Dislocation
- Implant loosening/subsidence/osteolysis
- Periprosthetic fractures
- Implant failure.

Hemorrhage and Hematoma Formation

Patients on blood thinners and certain medical diseases like hemophilia/blood dyscrasias are prone to excessive bleeding. Patients on salicylates and anti-inflammatory drugs also tend to bleed more. Hematomas are commoner with bony osteotomy. Bony bleed can be controlled partially by bone wax. Hemostasis should be achieved before closure. A suction drain deep to the fascia evacuates any bleeeding. This is usually removed after 24 hours. The objective of all these precautions is to prevent infection. Tranexamic acid given around surgery time is useful in controlling post-operative bleeding.

Infections

Infection of a total hip arthroplasty is a grave complication (Fig. 11.1). Current incidence is about 1% in primary arthroplasty. The predisposing factors are age; poor nutrition; co-morbidities like diabetes, rheumatoid arthritis, chronic urinary tract infection; patients on immunosuppressive drugs or steroids; previous surgeries; poor local skin condition, and post-operative hematoma.

Antibiotic prophylaxis and surgical asepsis are important factor in reducing the incidence. Most total hip infections are caused by Gram-positive organisms, e.g. *Staphylococcus aureus* and *S. epidermidis*.

Fitzgerald classified postoperative infections after total hip arthroplasty into three stages:
- Stage I infections occur in the immediate postoperative period (first 12 weeks).
- Stage II infections are deep delayed infections, which are indolent (from 3 to 24 months after surgery).
- Stage III or late infections are hematogenous (occur 2 years or longer after surgery).

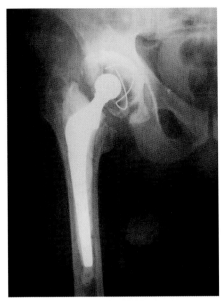

Fig. 11.1: Infected THR-radiograph

The treatment options for infected total hip arthroplasties consist of:
* Antibiotic therapy
* Incision and drainage of the hip
* Debridement and modified Girdlestone resection arthroplasty
* One or two-stage revision to a total hip arthroplasty (Figs 11.2A to C).

In stage I infections the patient presents with pain and swelling around the hip with fever, raised local temperature and the hip is painful, tender, erythematous and may drain spontaneously. Rising trend of blood parameters like TLC, DLC and C-reactive protein (Quantative) are suggestive of infection. Radiolucency with scalloping of the endosteal surface of the femur or acetabulum and some subperiosteal new bone may be seen after few weeks. A positive gallium 67 scan or indium 111 scan can be of value in identifying an infection (Fig. 11.3). If the infection is thought to be superficial the joint is not aspirated. The superficial layers of tissue are opened down to the deep fascia, in the operation theatre. A through irrigation and debridement is done. In case of doubt of infection involving the hip joint it is aspirated. If the infection extends deeper to the hip joint, the wound is opened further and thorough debridement and irrigation done. Cultures of fluid and tissues are taken and tissue specimens sent for histological study. Methylmethacrylate beads containing a broad-spectrum antibiotic may be placed in the wound. The appropriate antibiotic, as determined by the antibiotic sensitivity tests, is given intravenously for 4 to 6 weeks, depending on the healing of the wound and blood parameters. The prognosis is guarded. The infection may recur which may require removal of the components and cement.

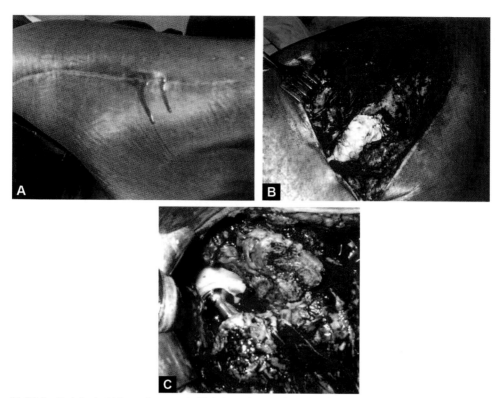

Figs 11.2A to C: *Infected hip replacement*: (A) Infected operative site, (B) Debrided and antibiotic loaded bone cement spacer inserted in 1st stage, (C) Revision hip surgery done once infection is controlled under the cover of parenteral antibiotics (2nd stage)

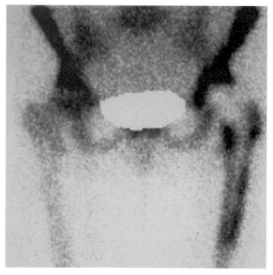

Fig. 11.3: *Bone scan infective hip*: Bone scan showing diffuse uptake around the femoral prosthesis, suggestive of infection; however, this may also be seen in aseptic loosening

Delayed infections may be acute or low-grade and chronic. Persistent, unexplained pain is suggestive of indolent infection. Pain may be dull and present both at rest and on weight-bearing. Persistent or intermittent wound drainage may be present. Fever may be absent and the white blood cell count may be normal. The serum C-reactive protein (Quantative) level is raised. A new bone formation or a localized scalloping of endosteal bone, erosion, loosening or progressing radiolucencies on radiographs is suggestive of infection. These findings may also be present with aseptic loosening however periosteal new bone formation is seen in infection. Indium 111–labeled WBC radionuclide scan is most reliable to detect infections. The hip joint is aspirated and fluid sent for examination. Deep delayed infections require removal of the implants with all of the cement extracted completely. Granulation and avascular tissues are excised. Antibiotic-impregnated methylmethacrylate beads or spacers are used for local antibiotic delivery. The wound is closed with interrupted sutures over suction drains.

Hematogenous spread is usually the cause of infection involving the total hip arthroplasty site at two years or later (Stage III). The focus may be an infected tooth, respiratory, genitourinary or skin infection. Patients with total hip arthroplasty therefore need to take antibiotic management immediately if they have a pyogenic infection. The diagnostic steps and treatment are the same as for delayed deep infection.

These patients may learn to live with Girdlestone excision arthroplasty or may undergo revision total hip arthroplasty. The revision may be a single stage procedure done at the time of initial debridement or preferrably a two stage procedure (Figs 11.2A to C). The debridement is done in the first stage and implantation of prosthesis in the 2nd stage. Treatment of the infection takes precedence over reconstruction of the hip. In a very rare case disarticulation of the hip may be indicated as a lifesaving measure because of uncontrollable infection or vascular complications.

Nerve Injuries

The sciatic, femoral, peroneal and obturator nerves can be injured depending on the approach used. This may be a direct surgical trauma, traction, pressure from retractors, extremity positioning, limb lengthening or thermal or pressure injury from cement. The incidence of nerve injuries reported in the literature is 0.7% to 3.5% in primary arthroplasties. Per operative lengthening may also lead to sciatic/peroneal nerve paresis or palsy. Sciatic nerve palsy may also occur as a result of subgluteal hematoma. Postoperative dislocation is another cause of sciatic nerve injury. Abduction pillows secured to the extremity with straps over the region of the fibular neck can cause peroneal nerve compression.

Vascular Injuries

Vascular injuries following primary total hip arthroplasty are rare (0.2% to 0.3%); however these may be grave injuries threatening the survival of the limb and the patient. The measures normally taken to avoid injury to the femoral nerve also protect the accompanying femoral artery and vein. The use of screws for acetabular socket fixation place the pelvic vessels at risk for injury. The use of a short drill bit and careful technique is mandatory whenever screws are to be placed in the anterior quadrants. Screw placement should be limited to the posterior quadrants wherever possible.

Urinary Tract Complications

Bladder infection is the most common complication involving the urinary tract, and the incidence is 7% to 14% after total hip arthroplasty. If routine urinalysis is suspect bacterial cultures and sensitivity tests should be obtained. If bladder infection is confirmed, the surgery should be delayed. Any recurrent infection after surgery should be treated immediately. Administration of prophylactic antibiotics (against Gram-negative organisms) is recommended. If the bladder is catheterized aseptic precautions should be taken to avoid infection, and prophylactic antibiotics started. An indwelling catheter beyond 48 hours increases the incidence of bladder infection. In male patients who develop postoperative urinary tract obstruction, prostatic surgery is delayed preferrably for 6 weeks or more and during this interval the patient should receive appropriate antibiotics.

Thrombo-embolism

Thrombo-embolic disease is the most common serious complication arising from total hip arthroplasty. It is the most common cause of death occurring within 3 months of surgery (Fig. 11.4). Thrombi in the calf alone, previously not thought to cause pulmonary emboli are now known to have proximal propagation. The risk of developing deep vein thrombosis may be present for a period of 3 weeks after surgery. Deep vein thrombosis also can lead to

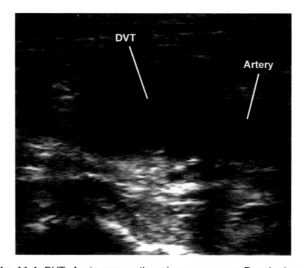

Fig. 11.4: DVT: Acute venous thrombus as seen on Doppler image

postphlebitic syndrome in the lower extremities. Several factors increase the risk of thromboembolism: (1) prior episode of thrombo-embolism, (2) prior venous surgery and varicose veins, (3) previous orthopedic operations, (4) advanced age, (5) malignancy, (6) congestive heart failure and chronic lower extremity swelling, (7) immobilization, (8) obesity and (9) use of oral contraceptives and hormones. The clinical diagnosis of deep vein thrombosis usually is made on the basis of pain and tenderness in the calf and thigh, positive Homans sign, unilateral swelling and erythema of the leg, low-grade fever, and rapid pulse. However, the diagnosis may not be clinically apparent. Doppler ultrasonography, however, is non invasive and can be easily repeated. It is not as helpful in diagnosis of calf thrombi and is observer dependant. None of these detect pelvic thrombi. The diagnosis of pulmonary embolism is based on symptoms of chest pain (especially if pleuritic in nature), evaluation by electrocardiogram and chest radiographs, and determination of arterial blood gas levels. Most pulmonary emboli are not clinically apparent. Venography is the gold standard for both calf and thigh thromboses. It is usually confirmed by radionuclide ventilation-perfusion lung scanning. D-dimer has a negative predictive value.

Currently both mechanical and pharmacological modalities are used for prophylaxis of thrombo-embolism. Pharmacological prophylaxis is used in almost all patients. Those most commonly used are low-molecular-weight heparins (LMWH) and aspirin. Low molecular weight heparin, e.g. Enoxaparin are used. However, there is a risk of epidural hematoma formation when used in conjunction with neuraxial anesthetics, especially with indwelling epidural catheters. The American protocol entails initiating thrombo-prophylaxis a night prior 12 hrs before the surgery omitting the morning dose. The European protocol recommends starting LMWH 12 hrs after the surgery. Aspirin although safe and inexpensive has been largely ineffective in preventing postoperative thrombo-embolism, when used alone. Some investigators have recommended continuing anticoagulants for 6 weeks after surgery.

Limb Length Discrepancy

Ideally, the leg lengths should be equal after total hip arthroplasty. However the patient should know before surgery that no assurance can be given about limb length equality (Fig. 11.5). If limb length discrepancy provides a stable hip, it is preferable to the risk of recurrent dislocation. Discrepancy of less than 1 cm generally is well tolerated. If lengthening exceeds 2.5 cm, sciatic palsy may result. The risk of excessive limb lengthening can be minimized by a combination of careful preoperative planning and operative technique. Use of a prosthesis that will allow intraoperative restoration of both limb length and femoral offset is recommended. The changes on the acetabular side of the joint may add to the limb length discrepancy.

Dislocation

The average incidence of dislocation after total hip arthroplasty is approximately 3% (Fig. 11.6). Factors contributing to this risk include (1) previous hip surgery or revision total

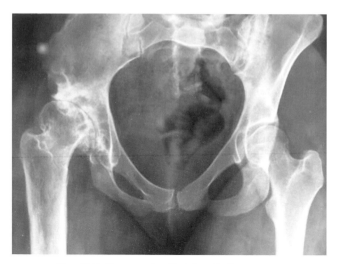

Fig. 11.5: Preoperative limb length discrepancy

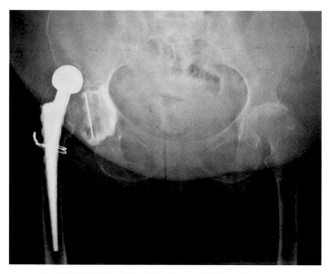

Fig. 11.6: Dislocation following total hip replacement

hip replacement, (2) a posterior surgical approach, (3) faulty positioning of one or both components, (4) impingement of the femur on the pelvis, residual osteophytes, the margin of the socket or protruded bone cement, (5) inadequate soft tissue tension or weak abductor muscles, (6) avulsion or nonunion of the greater trochanter, and (7) noncompliance or extremes of positioning in the peri-operative period.

Stability with trial implants should be checked before seating the final implant. Acetabular components with modular liners that have elevations may improve stability, but they may have the opposite effect if it is rotated into an inappropriate orientation. Paramedics and other attendants of the patient should be aware of the positions likely to cause dislocation. These may differ from patient to patient.

A dislocated total hip can be reduced gently to minimize damage to the articulating surfaces under intravenous sedation and analgesia. General anesthesia may be required for closed/open reduction. Image intensification is useful. Modular polyethylene liners may dissociate from their metal backings. Joint reduction is followed by a period of bed rest in abduction; traction or immobilization for 6 weeks to 3 months.

If dislocation becomes recurrent, revision surgery is usually required. If instability is compounded by neurological deficit or abductor insufficiency, revision to a bipolar prosthesis may be considered. Alternatively, a constrained socket design may be used.

Thigh Pain and Periprosthetic Fractures

Thigh pain is a complication seen following cementless total hip replacement, more commonly with extensively porous coated femoral stems. Thigh pain may rarely be a harbinger of periprosthetic femoral fracture (Fig. 11.7). Peri-prosthetic fractures are more common on the femoral side and usually require some treatment viz fixation or revision surgery. Acetabular fractures also are commoner than recognized but may not be clinically apparent. The predisposing factors for femoral fractures are osteoporosis, cortical defects from previous surgery or fixation devices, complex deformities of the proximal femur and breach during broaching or insertion of the femoral component.

Prophylactic placement of cerclage wires should be considered when the cortex is thin or has been weakened or has stress risers. Postoperative femoral shaft fractures may occur

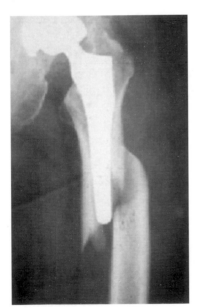

months or years after surgery, mostly near the tip of the stem or proximal to it. The treatment of periprosthetic femoral fractures include traction; open reduction and internal fixation of the fracture while leaving the stem in situ or femoral revision with or without adjunctive internal fixation depending on the level of fracture.

Osteolysis, Aseptic Loosening and Stem Failure

Femoral and acetabular loosening and osteolysis have emerged as the most serious long-term complications of total hip arthroplasty and the most common indications for revision (Fig. 11.8). In all patients suspected of having loosening the possibility of infection must be considered. Initially osteolysis was attributed to particulate methamethylcrylate debris and was called the cement

Fig. 11.7: Periprosthetic fracture of shaft femur

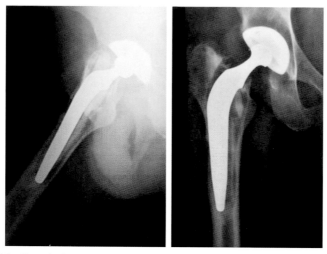

Fig. 11.8: *Osteolysis and aseptic loosening:* Significant loosening of femoral stem

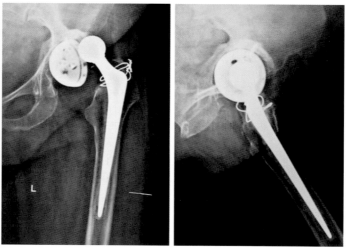

Fig. 11.9: *Osteolysis and aseptic loosening:* Osteolysis around both acetabular and femoral components with subluxation of the joint because of consequent implant malpositioning

disease. The final pathway however, appears to be related to the host response to particulate debris of all types. Therefore the general term osteolysis is more appropriate. In cementless fixation like the cemented implants particles of polyethylene and other debris are dispensed through the joint fluid, and any area of bone accessed by joint fluid is a potential site for deposition of debris and osteolysis. Many patients with acetabular osteolysis remain asymptomatic until catastrophic failure occurs from gross implant migration or periprosthetic fracture. Hence serial radiographs must be done regularly for the development of osteolysis and lytic changes. Loose implants and large lytic lesions are clear indications for surgery (Fig. 11.9).

Establishing whether symptoms are the result of aseptic loosening or infection can be difficult. The diagnosis of loosening is accepted in most instances if the radiolucent zone about one or both components is 2 mm or more in width and a patient has symptoms on weight-bearing and motion that are relieved by rest. In cement-less acetabular component socket migration, screw breakage, fracture of the metal shell, and defoliation of the porous surface are evidence of loosening. A continuous radiolucent line may indicate stable fibrous in-growth and may be compatible with a successful clinical result. On the femoral side, late subsidence or migration, separation of porous surfaces, and component fracture are evidence of loosening. Divergent sclerotic lines indicate axial or rotational instability.

Deformation and fracture of the stem occur in response to cyclic loading and usually develop several years after surgery. The treatment is revision total hip arthroplasty.

Miscellaneous

Postoperative heterotopic ossification varies in amount. It develops most commonly in men and in patients who have been operated upon because of ankylosing spondylitis, etc. Direct lateral approach has as lightly higher incidence of heterotopic ossification. The incidence is about 13% in the western literature. It usually is painless but may restrict motion to varying extents. The current medicines used for prevention of heterotopic bone are low-dose radiation and indomethacin.

There have been isolated reports of fat embolism syndrome occurring after total hip arthroplasty. Venting of the canal and pulsatile lavage to remove marrow elements, slow introduction of the femoral component aid in reducing the amount of embolic debris.

Trochanteric osteotomy, now rarely done, has an incidence of nonunion from 3% to 8%. Stable fibrous union without proximal migration usually produces good functional results with little pain. Migration of more than 2 cm significantly impairs abductor function and has an increased incidence of dislocation requires trochanteric repair.

Chapter Twelve

Newer Advances in
Hip Arthroplasty

Technology in hip arthroplasty is rapidly evolving. All of this is directed to improve the life span and function of the join, to enable the patient lead a near normal lifestyle.

The attempts are mult-pronged aimed at:

- Improving the longevity of acetabular and femoral stem fixation.
- Improving the durability and smoothness of the bearing surfaces.
- Increasing the stability and arc of movement at hip joint.
- To decrease the size of the primary implant.
- To decrease the size of incision to enable early healing and recovery.
- To achieve perfect orientation of the prosthesis at the time of initial fixation.

Lot of work is going on to achieve all this.

The factor in hip replacement reducing the life of implant has been the wear of the polyethylene over time, through the millions of cycles that the patients put their hips through normal activities of daily living. Recent advances in bearing surface technology has evolved a new generation of alternative bearing surfaces that are more resistant to wear and will hopefully allow hip replacements last even longer, especially in younger patients who require hip replacement surgery. The alternative bearings consist of highly cross-linked polyethylene, ceramics and all-metal bearing couples. These new materials are more resistant to wear than traditional polyethylene and are expected to give longer life to the bearing ends and also reduce the chance of debris induced osteolysis and implant loosening (Fig. 12.1).

In recent years, there has been a re-emergence of **resurfacing hip arthroplasty** (Fig. 12.2). This procedure is indicated for relatively younger patients with degenerative hip joint diseases, when conservative measures have failed. The current evidence for the clinical and cost effectiveness of hip resurfacing arthroplasty is principally in individuals less than 65 years of age. Current resurfacing techniques use metal on metal components (cobalt-

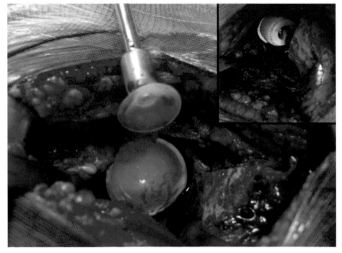

Fig. 12.1: Ceramic-on-ceramic hip: These have extremely low wear-rate

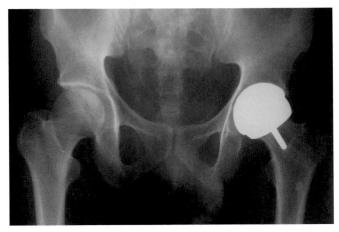

Fig. 12.2: *Surface replacement*. Surface replacement restores the anatomy of the hip without damaging much of the bone stock. Large bearing gives a larger range of motion.

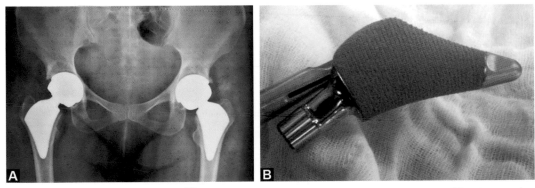

Figs 12.3A and B: Mini hip. Proxima™ hip is a mini hip which makes revision surgery easy. The stem can be attached to heads of various types viz. metal, ceramics and sizes

chromium-molybdenum alloy) and involve minimal bone resection. Proponents suggest that the procedure will restore normal anatomy, maximize proprioception, minimize dislocation rates, and will be amenable to easy revision should it fail in the future.

In patients where the femoral head cannot be preserved **smaller designs of femoral stems** have been made, e.g. the Proxima™ Hip (J & J, DePuy) (Fig. 12.3), which make revision surgeries less extensive. The newer design of modular femoral stems can be mated with femoral heads of various sizes and types allowing better on-table options to the operating

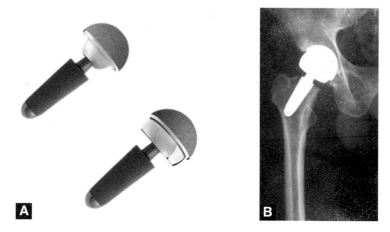

Figs 12.4A and B: (A) Cigar stem™ (B) Postoperative X-ray of Cigar stem™

surgeon. These heads may also be revised without exchanging the stems while performing revision surgeries. Cigar stem is another new design of a mini-hip replacement (Fig. 12.4).

To improve patients' outcome and shorten the hospital stay, orthopedic surgeons are exploring the option of **mini-invasive total hip arthroplasty**. This potentially helps to reduce complication rate, decrease blood loss, reduce early postoperative pain, accelerate rehabilitation, and provide a more attractive appearance. However, recent reports have highlighted that a shorter incision can increase the risk of peri-operative complication. At the same time, studies show no difference in early rehabilitation and hospital stay between patients undergoing mini-incision and standard incision total hip arthroplasty. Also that it is technically more difficult to achieve an optimal prosthesis placement because of a restricted visual field. Furthermore damage to neuro-vascular structure, to prosthetic surface during implantation and longer operative times are definite risks. This may be a single incision or two incision technique. Patient selection is important, a thin built, non-muscular female patient is an ideal candidate. Techniques not requiring transection of tendon or muscle (two incision technique) enable early recovery. Special instrumentation with C-arm assistance enable accurate component alignment and position. This technique requires meticulous knowledge of hip anatomy and specialized surgical training in the field.

The use of **computer assisted surgery (CAS)** (Fig. 12.5) is to optimize the placement of the prosthesis. This is a useful adjunct to minimally invasive surgery. The surgeon can achieve perfect implant alignment and positioning using CAS. Alignment errors are associated with rapid surface wear, implant failure and less satisfactory functional results.

Structural allografts both acetabular and femoral are being used to augment bone stock in revision surgeries. These allograft-prosthetic composite enhances longevity of the procedure and also helps in better attachment of host bone (especially greater trochanter)

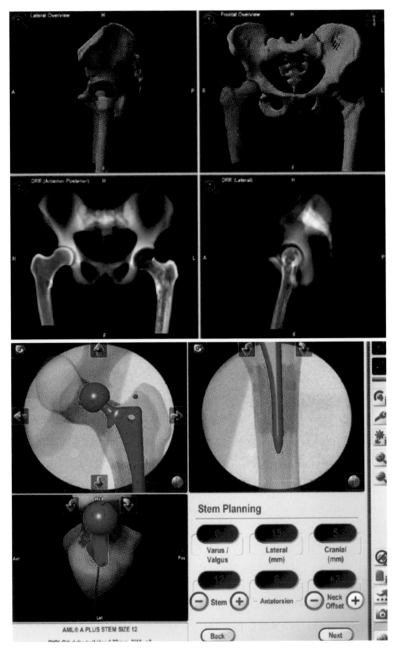

Fig. 12.5: Computer assisted surgeries. Computer navigation makes planning easy and execution more reliable and predictable

and muscles to the construct, however there is a risk of non-union, disease transmission, graft resorption and local infection. Successful allografting facilitates subsequent revision surgery, if need be.

Instrumentation in Hip Replacement Surgery

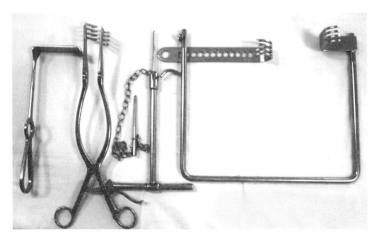

Various retractors used in hip surgeries: Deep Langenbach retractor, mastoid type retractor, pin retractor, Charnley type retractor

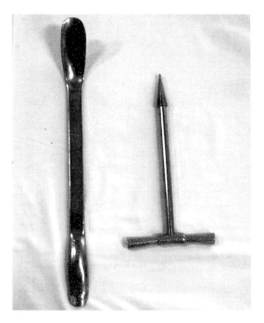

Instruments for dislocation or removal of femoral head: Murphy's skid, myomectomy screw (Judet extractor)

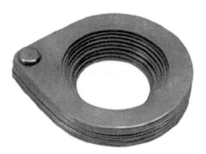

Femoral head gauge

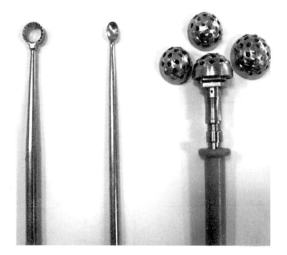

Instruments for acetabular preparation: Ring curette; long curette (also used on the femoral side), acetabular reamers with handle

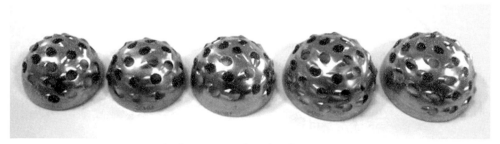

Acetabular reamer heads of various sizes

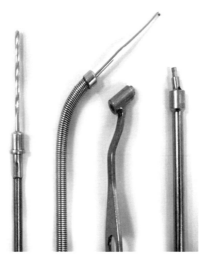

Instruments for acetabular screw fixation: Drill bit, depth gauge, drill guide, screw driver

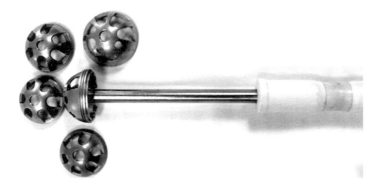

Trial acetabular cups: Various sizes; with handle

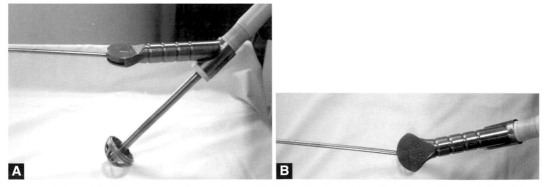

Cup holder with the anteversion guide: (A) The pin should point the ipsilateral shoulder. (B) The desired anteversion may be set accordingly we prefer 10 degrees of anteversion

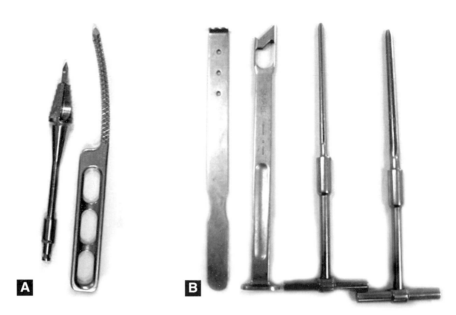

Instruments for femoral canal preparation: (A) Starting reamer and lateral broach (B) Trochanteric lever, box chisel (anteversion osteotome), straight reamers (two sizes).

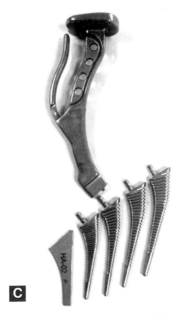

Instruments for femoral canal preparation: (C) Reamers with handle and neck osteotomy guide on the left end (for Corail™ cementless stem)

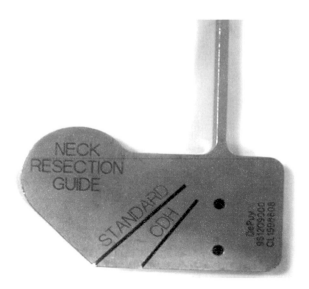

Femoral neck osteotomy guide: For C-stem™ instrumentation cemented prosthesis

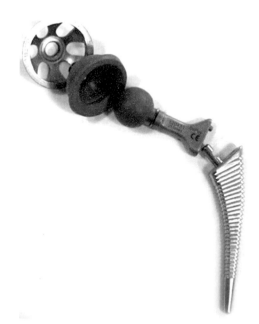

Complete cementless assembly: Metallic shell with trial liner,
trial head, trial neck and stem (Broach)

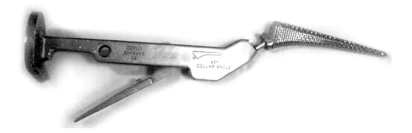

Broach for cemented stem with handle

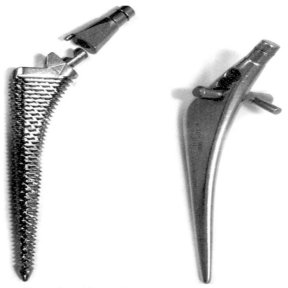

Cemented trial stem: Broach with neck attachment as trial cemented femoral stem. Trial femoral stem (C-Stem™) with adjustment for neck length

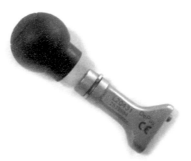

Trial prosthetic femoral head (extra-long, note the skirting) with trial neck